Food

Harnessing the Healing Power of Nutrition

Grace Hamilton

Food as Medicine

© Copyright 2024 by *Grace Hamilton*

All rights reserved

Table of Contents

Chapter 1: Understanding the Healing Properties of Food

Nutrients and Their Therapeutic Roles

Nutrients play an indispensable role in maintaining health and preventing diseases. These essential substances are the building blocks of life, fueling our bodies with energy and supporting critical physiological functions. Each nutrient carries its own unique therapeutic properties, and understanding these can transform how we approach food and health.

Proteins, carbohydrates, and fats are the primary macronutrients that provide energy and are crucial for bodily functions. Proteins, composed of amino acids, are vital for growth, repair, and maintenance of tissues. They play an essential role in producing enzymes, hormones, and neurotransmitters, which are crucial for communication within the body. High-quality protein sources, such as lean meats, fish, eggs, and legumes, offer the amino acids necessary for optimal physical and mental health.

Carbohydrates are the body's main energy source, providing fuel for both the brain and muscles. Complex carbohydrates, found in whole grains, vegetables, and fruits, are particularly beneficial as they are digested slowly, providing a steady release of energy. They also contain fiber, which aids in digestion, helps regulate blood sugar levels, and supports cardiovascular health by lowering cholesterol.

Fats, often misunderstood, are essential for various bodily functions. They are a concentrated energy source and are necessary for the absorption of fat-soluble vitamins like A, D, E, and K. Healthy fats, such as those found in avocados, nuts, seeds, and olive oil, support brain health, reduce inflammation, and protect against heart disease. Omega-3 and omega-6 fatty acids, specific types of polyunsaturated fats, are particularly crucial as they have anti-inflammatory properties and are linked to improved cardiovascular health and cognitive function.

Vitamins and minerals, although required in smaller quantities, are no less critical. These micronutrients play a myriad of roles in maintaining health. For instance, vitamin C is a powerful antioxidant that supports the immune system, promotes skin health, and aids in the absorption of iron. Found in citrus fruits, strawberries, and bell peppers, vitamin C is also vital in the synthesis of collagen, a protein that maintains skin elasticity and wound healing.

Vitamin D, often called the "sunshine vitamin," is crucial for bone health as it aids in calcium absorption. It also plays a role in immune function and inflammation regulation. While our bodies can synthesize vitamin D through sunlight exposure, dietary sources like fatty fish, fortified dairy products, and mushrooms can help ensure adequate intake, especially in individuals with limited sun exposure.

Minerals such as calcium, magnesium, and potassium are equally important. Calcium is well-known for its role in bone and teeth health, but it also supports muscle function and nerve transmission. Dairy products, leafy greens, and fortified plant milks are excellent sources of calcium. Magnesium, involved in over 300 biochemical reactions in the body, supports muscle and nerve function, regulates blood sugar levels, and contributes to bone health. Nuts, seeds, and whole grains are rich in magnesium. Potassium, found in bananas, potatoes, and legumes, helps maintain fluid balance, supports muscle contractions, and reduces the risk of hypertension by counterbalancing the effects of sodium.

The therapeutic roles of nutrients extend beyond their basic functions, reaching into the realm of disease prevention and management. For instance, antioxidants, found in many vitamins and phytochemicals, neutralize free radicals, reducing oxidative stress and lowering the risk of chronic diseases such as cancer, cardiovascular disease, and neurodegenerative disorders. Foods rich in antioxidants include berries, nuts, dark chocolate, and green tea.

Phytochemicals, naturally occurring compounds in plants, offer additional health benefits. These bioactive substances, such as flavonoids, carotenoids, and polyphenols, have been shown to possess anti-inflammatory, anti-cancer, and heart-protective properties. Consuming a diet rich in colorful fruits and vegetables ensures a diverse intake of these potent compounds.

Moreover, certain nutrients have been linked to mental health benefits. Omega-3 fatty acids, for example, are associated with reduced symptoms of depression and anxiety. B vitamins, including folate and B12, are crucial for brain health and have been implicated in reducing the risk of cognitive decline and mood disorders. Leafy greens, beans, and fortified cereals provide these essential vitamins.

The relationship between nutrients and health is deeply interconnected, and deficiencies can lead to a host of health issues. For instance, iron deficiency can result in anemia, characterized by fatigue and weakened immunity. Ensuring adequate intake of iron-rich foods like red meat, beans, and spinach can prevent this condition. Similarly, insufficient vitamin B12 can lead to neurological issues and pernicious anemia, highlighting the importance of consuming animal products or fortified foods for those at risk.

Understanding the therapeutic roles of nutrients empowers individuals to make informed dietary choices that support their health and well-being. By prioritizing a balanced diet rich in whole foods, one can harness the healing potential of nutrients to prevent disease, support recovery, and maintain optimal health.

Adopting a nutrient-dense diet not only satisfies the body's basic nutritional needs but also provides a foundation for lifelong health. This approach emphasizes the consumption of a variety of foods, each offering a unique combination of nutrients that work synergistically to promote health. Embracing a diverse array of foods ensures that the body receives a broad spectrum of nutrients, reducing the likelihood of deficiencies and supporting overall well-being.

Incorporating these principles into daily life can be as simple as choosing whole, unprocessed foods over refined options, focusing on colorful fruits and vegetables, and being mindful of portion sizes to maintain a balanced intake. By recognizing the therapeutic roles of nutrients, individuals can transform their approach to eating, viewing food as a powerful tool for health and healing rather than merely a source of sustenance. In doing so, they take an active role in their own health journey, laying the groundwork for a vibrant and fulfilling life.

Antioxidants and Their Impact on Health

Antioxidants are nature's powerful defenders against the wear and tear of daily life. These compounds, found abundantly in a variety of foods, play a crucial role in maintaining health by combating oxidative stress. Oxidative stress occurs when there is an imbalance between free radicals—molecules with unpaired electrons that can cause cellular damage—and the body's ability to neutralize them with antioxidants. This imbalance has been linked to a range of chronic diseases, including cancer, cardiovascular disorders, and neurodegenerative conditions.

Free radicals are a natural byproduct of metabolic processes, but they can also be generated by external factors such as pollution, radiation, and cigarette smoke. The human body is equipped with a complex antioxidant defense system, including enzymes and small molecules, to counteract these reactive species. However, to bolster this defense system, a diet rich in antioxidants is essential.

Antioxidants neutralize free radicals by donating an electron, thus preventing them from causing cellular damage. This protective mechanism is vital for preserving the integrity of DNA, proteins, and lipids, which are susceptible to oxidative harm. By safeguarding these cellular components, antioxidants contribute to the prevention of mutations that can lead to cancer, the stabilization of cell membranes, and the protection of essential cellular functions.

One of the most well-known antioxidants is vitamin C, which is highly effective in protecting against oxidative damage. It is involved in regenerating other antioxidants, such as vitamin E, and is crucial for collagen synthesis and immune function. Foods rich in vitamin C, including citrus fruits, kiwi, and bell peppers, can enhance the body's antioxidant capacity.

Vitamin E, another potent antioxidant, protects cell membranes from oxidative damage by reacting with lipid radicals. This fat-soluble vitamin is found in nuts, seeds, and vegetable oils, and it supports skin health and immune function. Its role in preventing lipid oxidation is particularly important in reducing the risk of cardiovascular diseases.

Beta-carotene, a precursor to vitamin A, is another antioxidant with significant health benefits. It neutralizes free radicals and supports immune function and eye health. Beta-carotene is abundant in orange and yellow fruits and vegetables such as carrots, sweet potatoes, and apricots.

Polyphenols, a diverse group of antioxidants found in plant foods, are known for their health-promoting properties. These compounds, including flavonoids, tannins, and lignans, have been linked to reduced inflammation, improved vascular health, and a lower risk of chronic diseases. Tea, coffee, berries, and dark chocolate are rich sources of polyphenols that can be easily incorporated into the diet.

Flavonoids, a subgroup of polyphenols, are particularly noteworthy for their role in cardiovascular health. They support the production of nitric oxide, a molecule that helps relax blood vessels and improve circulation. This action reduces blood pressure and improves overall heart health. Berries, onions, and apples are excellent sources of flavonoids.

Resveratrol, a polyphenol found in red wine and grapes, has gained attention for its potential anti-aging properties. It activates certain genes associated with longevity and cellular repair, offering protective effects against age-related diseases. While moderate red wine consumption can be part of a healthy diet, resveratrol supplements are also available for those seeking its benefits without alcohol intake.

Antioxidants also play a crucial role in brain health. The brain is particularly vulnerable to oxidative stress due to its high oxygen consumption and lipid-rich environment. Antioxidants help protect neuronal integrity and support cognitive function. For example, the consumption of berries rich in anthocyanins has been linked to improved memory and reduced risk of neurodegenerative diseases.

Moreover, antioxidants have a significant impact on skin health. They protect against damage caused by ultraviolet (UV) radiation, pollution, and other environmental stressors. Vitamins C and E, along with other antioxidants found in fruits and vegetables, can enhance skin elasticity, reduce wrinkles, and promote a youthful appearance.

Incorporating antioxidant-rich foods into daily meals is a practical strategy for enhancing health and longevity. A diet abundant in colorful fruits and vegetables, whole grains, nuts, and seeds provides a diverse range of antioxidants that work synergistically to protect the body from oxidative damage.

Cooking methods can also influence the antioxidant content of foods. For instance, steaming and blanching vegetables can preserve their antioxidant properties better than boiling. Additionally, pairing foods rich in vitamins C and E can enhance their combined antioxidant effects, offering greater protection against free radicals.

While dietary supplements can provide additional antioxidants, obtaining these compounds from whole foods is generally recommended. Whole foods contain a complex array of nutrients and phytochemicals that work together to promote health. Supplements may be considered for individuals with specific dietary restrictions or increased nutritional needs.

Understanding the role of antioxidants in health underscores the importance of a balanced and varied diet. By prioritizing antioxidant-rich foods, individuals can take proactive steps toward reducing oxidative stress and its associated health risks. This approach not only supports overall well-being but also empowers individuals to harness the natural protective mechanisms of food in their pursuit of a healthier life.

The Role of Phytochemicals in Disease Prevention

Phytochemicals, the naturally occurring compounds found in plants, have captivated the attention of researchers and health enthusiasts alike with their potential to prevent and combat a myriad of diseases. These bioactive substances are responsible for the vibrant colors, flavors, and aromas of fruits, vegetables, herbs, and spices. Beyond their sensory appeal, phytochemicals are emerging as powerful allies in the fight against chronic illnesses, offering a promising avenue for disease prevention.

For centuries, traditional medicine systems around the world have harnessed the benefits of plant-derived compounds. Modern science is now unraveling the mechanisms behind these ancient practices, revealing a complex interplay between phytochemicals and human health. These compounds are not essential nutrients like vitamins and minerals, yet they exert significant biological effects that can influence health outcomes.

One of the most compelling roles of phytochemicals is their antioxidant activity. These compounds help neutralize free radicals, the unstable molecules that can cause cellular damage and contribute to chronic diseases such as cancer, cardiovascular disorders, and neurodegeneration. By protecting cells from oxidative stress, phytochemicals help maintain cellular integrity and function, reducing the risk of mutation and disease.

Among the myriad of phytochemicals, flavonoids are particularly noteworthy for their health-promoting properties. Found abundantly in fruits, vegetables, tea, and wine, flavonoids have been linked to reduced inflammation, improved heart health, and enhanced immune function. Their ability to modulate signaling pathways and gene expression positions them as influential players in disease prevention.

Carotenoids, another class of phytochemicals, are responsible for the red, orange, and yellow hues in foods like carrots, sweet potatoes, and tomatoes. These compounds, including beta-carotene, lutein, and lycopene, have been associated with a lower risk of certain cancers and eye diseases. Carotenoids' antioxidant properties, combined with their ability to modulate immune responses, make them valuable in protecting against age-related macular degeneration and other degenerative conditions.

The cruciferous vegetable family, which includes broccoli, cauliflower, and cabbage, is a rich source of glucosinolates. These sulfur-containing compounds have shown promise in cancer prevention due to their ability to inhibit the growth of cancer cells and promote their elimination. The consumption of cruciferous vegetables has been associated with a reduced risk of various cancers, including those of the lung, breast, and prostate.

Polyphenols, a diverse group of phytochemicals, are renowned for their anti-inflammatory and cardioprotective effects. Resveratrol, a polyphenol found in grapes and red wine, has gained attention for its potential role in longevity and cardiovascular health. It activates certain pathways that promote cellular repair and resilience, offering protection against heart disease and other age-related conditions.

The consumption of phytochemical-rich foods is linked to improved gut health, which plays a critical role in overall well-being. Phytochemicals can influence the composition and activity of the gut microbiota, the diverse community of microorganisms residing in the digestive tract. A balanced gut microbiota is essential for proper digestion, nutrient absorption, and immune function. Moreover, certain phytochemicals, such as those found in garlic and onions, possess prebiotic properties, promoting the growth of beneficial bacteria in the gut.

Phytochemicals also exhibit antimicrobial and antiviral properties, aiding the body's defense against infections. Compounds like allicin, found in garlic, and curcumin, present in turmeric, have been shown to inhibit the growth of harmful bacteria and viruses. These properties underscore the potential of phytochemicals as natural alternatives to synthetic antimicrobials in supporting immune health.

Incorporating a variety of phytochemical-rich foods into the diet is a practical strategy for harnessing their health benefits. A colorful plate, filled with an array of fruits, vegetables, whole grains, nuts, and seeds, ensures a diverse intake of these compounds. Emphasizing whole foods over processed ones helps preserve the integrity of phytochemicals, maximizing their protective effects.

Cooking methods can influence the bioavailability of phytochemicals. For instance, lightly steaming vegetables like broccoli can preserve glucosinolates, while cooking tomatoes enhances the availability of lycopene. Pairing certain foods can also enhance the absorption of phytochemicals, such as combining fat-rich foods with carotenoid-containing vegetables to improve bioavailability.

While dietary supplements containing isolated phytochemicals are available, whole foods offer a synergistic combination of nutrients and compounds that work together to promote health. The consumption of whole foods ensures a broader spectrum of phytochemicals and other beneficial nutrients, providing a more holistic approach to disease prevention.

The role of phytochemicals in disease prevention is a testament to the power of nature's pharmacy. By embracing a diet rich in plant-based foods, individuals can tap into the protective potential of these compounds, reducing the risk of chronic diseases and supporting overall health. The journey toward optimal health is paved with colorful, flavorful, and aromatic foods that nourish the body and delight the senses. Through the mindful selection of phytochemical-rich foods, individuals can embark on a path to wellness and vitality, reaping the rewards of nature's most potent defense against disease.

Anti-inflammatory Foods and Their Benefits

The body's inflammatory response is a crucial part of our immune defense, designed to protect us from infection and injury. However, when inflammation becomes chronic, it can contribute to a host of health issues, including arthritis, heart disease, diabetes, and even cancer. The food we consume plays a significant role in either exacerbating or mitigating inflammatory processes. Embracing a diet rich in anti-inflammatory foods can be a powerful strategy for promoting health and preventing disease.

Anti-inflammatory foods are characterized by their ability to reduce inflammation and oxidative stress within the body. These foods are typically high in antioxidants, omega-3 fatty acids, and other bioactive compounds that modulate inflammatory pathways. By incorporating these foods into daily meals, individuals can support their body's natural healing processes and reduce the risk of chronic inflammation-related conditions.

Fruits and vegetables are cornerstones of an anti-inflammatory diet. They are rich in vitamins, minerals, and phytochemicals that possess potent anti-inflammatory properties. Berries, such as blueberries, strawberries, and raspberries, are particularly noteworthy for their high content of anthocyanins, which have been shown to reduce inflammation and oxidative stress. Leafy greens like spinach, kale, and Swiss chard are abundant in antioxidants and polyphenols, compounds that can help lower inflammatory markers.

Cruciferous vegetables, including broccoli, cauliflower, and Brussels sprouts, contain glucosinolates, which are sulfur-containing compounds with anti-inflammatory and anti-cancer properties. These vegetables support the body's detoxification processes and promote the elimination of harmful substances that can trigger inflammation.

Omega-3 fatty acids, found in abundance in fatty fish such as salmon, mackerel, and sardines, are essential for combating inflammation. These healthy fats are integral components of cell membranes and play a role in the production of anti-inflammatory molecules. Regular consumption of omega-3-rich foods can help lower levels of inflammatory markers like C-reactive protein (CRP) and reduce the risk of chronic diseases.

Nuts and seeds, such as walnuts, flaxseeds, and chia seeds, are excellent plant-based sources of omega-3 fatty acids. They also provide a wealth of other nutrients, including fiber, protein, and magnesium, which contribute to overall health and well-being. Incorporating a variety of nuts and seeds into the diet can offer protective effects against inflammation and its associated health risks.

Spices and herbs, often overlooked in the realm of nutrition, are potent anti-inflammatory agents. Turmeric, renowned for its active compound curcumin, has been extensively studied for its ability to inhibit inflammatory pathways and reduce pain and swelling. Ginger, another powerful spice, contains gingerols and shogaols, compounds that possess anti-inflammatory and antioxidant effects. Regular use of these spices in cooking can enhance the flavor of dishes while offering therapeutic benefits.

Olive oil, a staple of the Mediterranean diet, is rich in monounsaturated fats and polyphenols that exhibit anti-inflammatory properties. Extra virgin olive oil, in particular, contains oleocanthal, a compound with effects similar to nonsteroidal anti-inflammatory drugs (NSAIDs). Using olive oil as a primary fat source can support heart health and reduce inflammation throughout the body.

Whole grains, such as oats, quinoa, and brown rice, are high in fiber and nutrients that can help lower inflammation. Unlike refined grains, whole grains retain their bran and germ, providing a rich source of essential nutrients and bioactive compounds. The fiber in whole grains aids in maintaining a healthy gut microbiota, which plays a crucial role in regulating inflammation and immune function.

Green tea, celebrated for its high concentration of catechins, offers anti-inflammatory and antioxidant benefits. Regular consumption of green tea has been associated with reduced risk of chronic diseases and improved markers of inflammation. Its bioactive compounds can help modulate inflammatory pathways and support cardiovascular health.

Adopting an anti-inflammatory diet involves more than just adding certain foods; it also requires reducing the intake of pro-inflammatory foods. Processed foods high in refined sugars, trans fats, and artificial additives can exacerbate inflammation and should be minimized. Instead, focusing on whole, unprocessed foods can provide the nutrients needed to support the body's natural defenses.

Hydration is another key component of an anti-inflammatory lifestyle. Drinking adequate water supports the body's detoxification processes and helps maintain optimal cellular function. Herbal teas and infused waters can also be included to promote hydration and provide additional antioxidants.

Incorporating anti-inflammatory foods into daily meals can be both simple and enjoyable. Starting the day with a breakfast of oatmeal topped with berries and walnuts provides a nutrient-dense, anti-inflammatory meal. For lunch, a salad with leafy greens, colorful vegetables, and a dressing made with olive oil and lemon delivers a variety of anti-inflammatory compounds. Dinner can feature fatty fish like salmon paired with roasted cruciferous vegetables and quinoa, offering a balanced and satisfying meal.

Snacks and beverages can also be opportunities to include anti-inflammatory foods. A handful of almonds or a green tea smoothie can provide a nutrient boost between meals. Incorporating spices like turmeric and ginger into soups, stews, and smoothies can further enhance their anti-inflammatory potential.

By prioritizing an anti-inflammatory diet, individuals can take proactive steps toward reducing the risk of chronic diseases and enhancing overall health. This approach not only supports the body's natural healing processes but also empowers individuals to make informed dietary choices that promote long-term well-being. Through mindful eating and the inclusion of a diverse array of anti-inflammatory foods, individuals can nurture their bodies and foster a foundation for a healthier, more vibrant life.

The Gut-Health Connection

The human gut is a bustling metropolis of activity, home to trillions of microorganisms collectively known as the gut microbiota. This complex ecosystem plays a crucial role in maintaining health, influencing everything from digestion and nutrient absorption to immune function and mental well-being. The connection between gut health and overall health is profound, and understanding this relationship opens the door to improved wellness through diet and lifestyle choices.

Central to the gut-health connection is the concept of balance. A diverse and balanced gut microbiota supports optimal digestion and protects against harmful pathogens. The gut serves as a barrier between the external environment and the bloodstream, and a well-functioning gut can effectively prevent the entry of harmful substances while allowing nutrients to pass through.

Diet is a primary factor that influences the composition and activity of the gut microbiota. A diet rich in fiber, prebiotics, and probiotics can promote a healthy gut environment. Fiber, found in fruits, vegetables, whole grains, and legumes, acts as a food source for beneficial bacteria. These bacteria ferment fiber into short-chain fatty acids, which have anti-inflammatory effects and support gut health.

Prebiotics are specific types of fiber that selectively nourish beneficial bacteria. Foods like garlic, onions, leeks, asparagus, and bananas are rich in prebiotics and can help increase the population of health-promoting bacteria in the gut. Regular consumption of prebiotic-rich foods can enhance microbial diversity and contribute to a balanced gut microbiota.

Probiotics, live beneficial bacteria found in fermented foods, can directly introduce healthy microbes into the gut. Yogurt, kefir, kimchi, sauerkraut, and miso are excellent sources of probiotics. These foods can help restore balance in the gut microbiota, especially after disruptions caused by antibiotics or illness.

The gut-brain axis is a bidirectional communication network that links the gut and the brain. This connection highlights the impact of gut health on mental and emotional well-being. The gut microbiota produces neurotransmitters, such as serotonin and dopamine, which are involved in mood regulation. An imbalance in gut bacteria has been associated with mental health conditions like depression and anxiety.

Stress and poor diet can disrupt the balance of the gut microbiota, leading to dysbiosis, a state where harmful bacteria outnumber beneficial ones. Dysbiosis is linked to a range of health issues, including digestive disorders, autoimmune diseases, and metabolic conditions. Addressing dysbiosis involves restoring balance through dietary changes, stress management, and possibly probiotics.

Immune function is intricately connected to gut health. A significant portion of the immune system resides in the gut, where it interacts with the microbiota to distinguish between harmful invaders and benign substances. A healthy gut microbiota supports the development and function of the immune system, enhancing the body's ability to fend off infections and diseases.

The gut barrier, composed of a single layer of epithelial cells, plays a critical role in maintaining health by preventing the entry of toxins and pathogens. Factors like poor diet, stress, and infections can compromise this barrier, leading to increased intestinal permeability, often referred to as "leaky gut." Leaky gut is associated with inflammation and the development of autoimmune conditions. Strengthening the gut barrier involves consuming a diet rich in anti-inflammatory foods, omega-3 fatty acids, and nutrients like zinc and vitamin D.

Incorporating fermented foods into meals is a practical way to support gut health. A breakfast of yogurt with fresh fruit and a sprinkle of flaxseeds provides probiotics, fiber, and prebiotics in one meal. For lunch, a salad with mixed greens, cherry tomatoes, avocado, and a side of sauerkraut offers a variety of nutrients and beneficial bacteria. Dinner can include a serving of grilled fish with a side of roasted vegetables and a miso soup, delivering omega-3 fatty acids and probiotics.

Hydration is essential for maintaining a healthy gut. Water supports digestion and helps flush out toxins. Herbal teas, such as ginger or peppermint, can aid digestion and soothe the gut. Limiting the intake of alcohol and caffeinated beverages can also support gut health by reducing irritation and inflammation.

Regular physical activity contributes to gut health by promoting diverse and balanced microbiota. Exercise can enhance the growth of beneficial bacteria and improve digestion. Finding enjoyable forms of movement, whether it's walking, yoga, or dancing, can support both physical and mental well-being.

Stress management is crucial for maintaining gut health. Chronic stress can negatively impact the gut-brain axis and alter the composition of the gut microbiota. Incorporating stress-reducing practices such as meditation, deep breathing, and mindfulness into daily routines can have a positive effect on gut health and overall wellness.

Listening to the body's hunger and fullness cues can promote mindful eating and support digestion. Eating slowly and savoring each bite allows the digestive system to function optimally and can prevent overeating. Paying attention to how different foods affect the body can guide dietary choices that promote gut health.

The journey to a healthy gut is a holistic one, involving dietary, lifestyle, and mental health considerations. By nurturing the gut microbiota through balanced nutrition, stress management, and mindful living, individuals can unlock the potential for improved health and vitality. This approach empowers individuals to take charge of their health, fostering a deeper connection between body and mind, and paving the way for a more vibrant and fulfilling life.

Chapter 2: Foods that Heal: A Comprehensive Guide

Superfoods and Their Nutritional Power

Superfoods have garnered a reputation for being nutritional powerhouses, offering a concentrated dose of vitamins, minerals, antioxidants, and other beneficial compounds. While no single food holds the key to perfect health, incorporating a variety of superfoods into one's diet can enhance overall well-being and vitality. These nutrient-dense foods are celebrated for their potential to boost energy, improve immune function, and support a healthy lifestyle.

One of the most renowned superfoods is the blueberry, a tiny fruit packed with antioxidants, particularly anthocyanins, which give it its deep blue color. These antioxidants help combat oxidative stress, reduce inflammation, and support brain health. Blueberries are also rich in vitamin C, vitamin K, and fiber, making them a versatile addition to smoothies, oatmeal, or salads.

Kale, a member of the cruciferous vegetable family, stands out for its impressive nutrient profile. This leafy green is loaded with vitamins A, C, and K, as well as calcium, potassium, and fiber. Kale's high content of antioxidants, including quercetin and kaempferol, contributes to its anti-inflammatory and heart-protective properties. Whether enjoyed raw in salads, sautéed as a side dish, or blended into green smoothies, kale is a versatile and nutritious choice.

Quinoa, an ancient grain revered by the Incas, has gained popularity as a superfood due to its unique nutritional composition. Unlike most plant-based foods, quinoa is a complete protein, containing all nine essential amino acids. It is also rich in fiber, magnesium, and iron, making it a valuable addition to vegetarian and vegan diets. Quinoa's mild flavor and fluffy texture make it a perfect base for salads, bowls, or breakfast porridge.

Chia seeds, tiny black seeds native to Central America, are celebrated for their high omega-3 fatty acid content. These essential fats support brain health, reduce inflammation, and promote heart health. Chia seeds are also an excellent source of fiber, protein, and calcium. When mixed with liquid, they form a gel-like consistency that can be used to thicken smoothies, make pudding, or replace eggs in baking recipes.

Avocado, often dubbed a superfood, is rich in healthy monounsaturated fats that support heart health and help absorb fat-soluble vitamins. This creamy fruit is also an excellent source of potassium, folate, and vitamins C, E, and K. Avocados can be enjoyed in a variety of ways, from spreading on toast to topping salads or blending into creamy sauces and dressings.

Salmon, a fatty fish known for its high omega-3 content, is a nutritional powerhouse that supports brain function, cardiovascular health, and inflammation reduction. Rich in high-quality protein, vitamin D, and selenium, salmon is an excellent choice for those seeking to boost their intake of essential nutrients. Grilled, baked, or poached, salmon pairs well with a variety of herbs and spices, making it a versatile and delicious option for any meal.

Turmeric, a vibrant yellow spice commonly used in Indian cuisine, has gained attention for its active compound, curcumin. Curcumin possesses potent anti-inflammatory and antioxidant properties, making turmeric a valuable addition to a health-conscious diet. Incorporating turmeric into dishes like curries, soups, or golden milk lattes can add flavor and nutrition while supporting overall health.

Almonds, nutrient-dense nuts, are an excellent source of healthy fats, protein, fiber, vitamin E, and magnesium. Regular consumption of almonds has been linked to improved heart health, weight management, and blood sugar control. Almonds can be enjoyed as a snack, added to trail mixes, or used as a base for homemade nut milk and butter.

Dark chocolate, with a cocoa content of 70% or higher, is not only a delicious treat but also a superfood rich in antioxidants, particularly flavonoids. These compounds support heart health, improve blood flow, and reduce inflammation. Enjoying a small piece of dark chocolate as part of a balanced diet can satisfy sweet cravings while providing health benefits.

Spirulina, a blue-green algae, is a superfood known for its high protein content and rich array of vitamins and minerals, including B vitamins, iron, and copper. Spirulina's antioxidants, including phycocyanin, have been shown to reduce inflammation and support immune function. Adding spirulina powder to smoothies, juices, or energy bars can boost nutrition and provide a natural energy lift.

Incorporating superfoods into a daily diet involves creativity and a willingness to experiment with new flavors and textures. Starting the day with a breakfast of oatmeal topped with blueberries, chia seeds, and a dollop of almond butter provides a nutrient-rich start. A lunch featuring a quinoa and kale salad with avocado and grilled salmon offers a balanced and satisfying meal. For dinner, a turmeric-infused curry with vegetables and brown rice delivers flavor and nutrition.

Snacks and beverages also present opportunities to include superfoods. A green smoothie with spinach, banana, almond milk, and spirulina makes a refreshing and energizing option. Dark chocolate-covered almonds or a homemade energy bar with nuts and seeds can provide a nutritious and satisfying treat.

While superfoods offer a wealth of nutrients, it's important to remember that they are not a cure-all. A balanced diet that includes a variety of whole foods, alongside a healthy lifestyle, is the foundation for optimal health. Superfoods can complement this approach by providing concentrated doses of essential nutrients that support overall well-being.

The journey toward incorporating superfoods into one's diet is an exciting exploration of flavors and nutrition. By embracing the diverse offerings of nature's bounty, individuals can enhance their health, boost their energy, and enjoy the delicious benefits of these nutritional powerhouses. Through mindful selection and preparation of superfoods, individuals can nourish their bodies and cultivate a more vibrant and fulfilling life.

The Benefits of Fermented and Probiotic-rich Foods

Fermented and probiotic-rich foods have been integral to human diets for centuries, cherished for their distinctive flavors and health-promoting properties. These foods undergo a natural process that not only preserves them but also enhances their nutritional value. By introducing beneficial bacteria into the gut, they support digestion, boost immunity, and contribute to overall well-being. Understanding the benefits of these foods offers a pathway to improved health and vitality.

The process of fermentation involves the breakdown of carbohydrates by microorganisms such as bacteria, yeast, and molds. This ancient preservation technique transforms simple ingredients into nutrient-rich foods with complex flavors and textures. Fermented foods are teeming with probiotics, live beneficial bacteria that populate the gut and support a healthy microbiome. A balanced gut microbiome is crucial for optimal digestion, nutrient absorption, and immune function.

Yogurt, one of the most popular fermented foods, is made by fermenting milk with specific bacterial cultures. This creamy and tangy dairy product is rich in calcium, protein, and probiotics. Regular consumption of yogurt can promote digestive health, enhance lactose digestion, and support a healthy weight. It is a versatile ingredient that can be enjoyed plain, sweetened with fruit, or used as a base for smoothies and dressings.

Kefir, a fermented milk drink, is similar to yogurt but contains a broader range of bacterial and yeast strains. This effervescent beverage is packed with probiotics, vitamins, and minerals. Kefir has been associated with improved digestion, enhanced immune response, and reduced inflammation. It can be consumed as a refreshing drink or used in recipes that call for buttermilk or yogurt.

Sauerkraut, made from fermented cabbage, is a staple in many traditional cuisines. This tangy and crunchy dish is rich in fiber, vitamins C and K, and probiotics. Sauerkraut supports digestion and gut health by providing beneficial bacteria that aid in breaking down food and absorbing nutrients. It pairs well with meats, sandwiches, and salads, adding a burst of flavor and nutrition.

Kimchi, a spicy Korean side dish, is made from fermented vegetables, typically cabbage and radishes, with a variety of seasonings. This flavorful dish is rich in vitamins, antioxidants, and probiotics. Kimchi consumption has been linked to improved digestive health, enhanced immune function, and lower cholesterol levels. It can be enjoyed as a condiment, side dish, or incorporated into soups and stews.

Miso, a traditional Japanese seasoning, is made by fermenting soybeans with salt and koji, a type of mold. This savory paste is rich in protein, vitamins, and minerals, and contains beneficial bacteria. Miso supports digestive health and provides a unique umami flavor to dishes. It can be used to make miso soup, marinades, or dressings, adding depth and richness.

Tempeh, a fermented soybean product, is a staple in Indonesian cuisine. This dense and nutty-flavored food is a complete protein, containing all essential amino acids. Tempeh is also rich in probiotics, fiber, and vitamins. It supports digestive health and provides a plant-based protein option for vegetarians and vegans. Tempeh can be sliced, marinated, and used in stir-fries, sandwiches, or salads.

Kombucha, a fermented tea beverage, is gaining popularity for its refreshing taste and health benefits. This effervescent drink is made by fermenting sweetened tea with a symbiotic culture of bacteria and yeast (SCOBY). Kombucha is rich in probiotics, antioxidants, and organic acids. It supports gut health, detoxification, and digestion. Available in various flavors, kombucha can be enjoyed as a healthful alternative to sugary sodas.

Incorporating fermented and probiotic-rich foods into the daily diet can have profound effects on gut health and overall well-being. These foods introduce a diverse array of beneficial bacteria to the gut, enhancing microbial diversity and balance. A healthy gut microbiome supports digestion, nutrient absorption, and immune function, while also influencing mood and mental health through the gut-brain axis.

The benefits of fermented foods extend beyond probiotics. The fermentation process increases the bioavailability of nutrients, making them more accessible to the body. It also reduces anti-nutrients like phytic acid, which can inhibit the absorption of minerals. As a result, fermented foods provide a concentrated source of vitamins, minerals, and antioxidants that support overall health.

For those new to fermented foods, starting with small portions and gradually increasing intake can help the body adjust to the influx of beneficial bacteria. This approach can minimize digestive discomfort and allow the gut to adapt to the changes. Experimenting with different types of fermented foods can add variety and excitement to meals, encouraging a more diverse and balanced diet.

Fermented foods can be easily incorporated into various meals and snacks. A breakfast of yogurt with fresh fruit and a sprinkle of granola provides a probiotic-rich start to the day. For lunch, a salad topped with kimchi or sauerkraut adds flavor and nutrition. Dinner can feature a miso-glazed fish or a tempeh stir-fry, offering a delicious and healthful meal. Snacks like kefir smoothies or a handful of cheese cubes can provide a probiotic boost between meals.

While fermented foods offer numerous health benefits, it is important to choose high-quality products with live and active cultures. Reading labels and selecting foods with minimal additives and preservatives can ensure optimal probiotic content. For those interested in home fermentation, making foods like sauerkraut, yogurt, or kombucha can be a rewarding and cost-effective way to enjoy these nutritious foods.

Incorporating fermented and probiotic-rich foods into the diet is a practical step toward enhancing gut health and overall wellness. By embracing these flavorful and nutrient-dense foods, individuals can support their digestive system, boost immunity, and cultivate a balanced and vibrant lifestyle. Through mindful selection and preparation of fermented foods, the path to improved health and vitality becomes both delicious and attainable.

Healing Herbs and Spices

Herbs and spices have long held a revered place in culinary and medicinal traditions around the world. These natural flavor enhancers not only add complexity and depth to dishes but also offer a wealth of health benefits. Their healing properties have been recognized for centuries, with many cultures incorporating them into remedies and treatments for various ailments. By weaving these aromatic wonders into daily life, one can harness their therapeutic potential and enrich both body and spirit.

Turmeric, with its vibrant golden hue, is one of the most celebrated spices in traditional medicine, particularly within Ayurvedic and Chinese practices. The key component of turmeric is curcumin, a powerful anti-inflammatory and antioxidant compound. Studies have shown that curcumin can help alleviate symptoms of arthritis, reduce inflammation, and support cognitive function. Incorporating turmeric into meals is as simple as adding it to soups, stews, or curries. For those seeking an extra boost, a warm cup of golden milk made with turmeric, milk (or plant-based alternative), and a dash of black pepper can be both soothing and health-promoting.

Ginger, known for its zesty and warming flavor, is another potent healing spice. Revered for its digestive benefits, ginger can alleviate nausea, reduce bloating, and support overall digestive health. Its anti-inflammatory properties also make it effective in relieving muscle pain and joint discomfort. Fresh ginger can be sliced and steeped in hot water for a calming tea, or grated into stir-fries, marinades, and baked goods for a punch of flavor. Combining ginger with honey and lemon creates a natural remedy for soothing sore throats and boosting immunity.

Cinnamon, with its sweet and woody aroma, has been used for centuries for both culinary and medicinal purposes. This versatile spice is rich in antioxidants and has anti-inflammatory and antimicrobial properties. Cinnamon can help regulate blood sugar levels, making it beneficial for individuals with insulin sensitivity or type 2 diabetes. Sprinkling cinnamon on oatmeal, adding it to smoothies, or incorporating it into baked goods can enhance flavor and provide health benefits. A cinnamon stick simmered in warm milk or tea can create a comforting and healthful beverage.

Garlic, a staple in kitchens worldwide, is renowned for its bold flavor and numerous health benefits. Rich in sulfur compounds, garlic has potent anti-inflammatory, antibacterial, and antiviral properties. Regular consumption of garlic can support heart health by reducing blood pressure and cholesterol levels. It also boosts the immune system, helping the body fend off infections. Fresh garlic can be minced and added to sauces, soups, and roasted vegetables. For those who enjoy its raw pungency, a garlic-infused olive oil can be a delightful addition to salads and dips.

Peppermint, with its refreshing menthol aroma, is a versatile herb used in both culinary and therapeutic contexts. Peppermint is known for its ability to soothe digestive issues, relieve headaches, and reduce nasal congestion. A cup of peppermint tea can provide relief from indigestion and promote relaxation. Fresh peppermint leaves can be added to salads, desserts, or infused in water for a refreshing twist. The essential oil, when diluted, can be applied topically to the temples for headache relief or inhaled to clear nasal passages.

Rosemary, an evergreen herb with a distinct pine-like fragrance, is celebrated for its cognitive-enhancing and antioxidant properties. Rosemary can improve memory, concentration, and overall brain function. It also supports digestion and has antimicrobial effects. Fresh or dried rosemary can be used to season roasted vegetables, meats, and soups, infusing dishes with its aromatic essence. A rosemary-infused olive oil can elevate the flavor of bread and salads. Additionally, inhaling the scent of rosemary essential oil can provide a natural mental boost.

Basil, beloved for its sweet and peppery flavor, is a staple in Mediterranean cooking. This aromatic herb is rich in antioxidants, anti-inflammatory compounds, and essential oils that support heart health and reduce oxidative stress. Fresh basil leaves can be used to make pesto, garnish salads, or flavor pasta dishes. Basil can also be infused into oils or vinegars for a flavorful and healthful addition to dressings and marinades. A simple basil tea, made by steeping fresh leaves in hot water, can offer a calming and aromatic experience.

Saffron, the precious spice derived from the Crocus sativus flower, is revered for its distinctive flavor and vibrant color. Saffron contains carotenoids and other bioactive compounds with antioxidant, anti-inflammatory, and mood-enhancing properties. It has been used in traditional medicine to support mood, alleviate symptoms of depression, and improve heart health. A small pinch of saffron can be steeped in warm milk or water to extract its flavor and color, then added to rice dishes, soups, and desserts for a luxurious touch.

Thyme, a fragrant herb with tiny leaves, is known for its antibacterial and antifungal properties. Thyme is rich in vitamins C and A, as well as thymol, a compound that supports respiratory health and boosts the immune system. Fresh or dried thyme can be used to season meats, vegetables, and stews, imparting a warm and earthy flavor. Thyme tea, made by steeping the leaves in hot water, can provide relief from coughs and colds. The essential oil, when diluted, can be used in steam inhalation to support respiratory health.

Incorporating healing herbs and spices into daily life is a simple yet powerful way to enhance health and well-being. These natural remedies can be used in cooking, brewed into teas, or applied topically in diluted essential oil form, offering a variety of ways to experience their benefits. Experimenting with different combinations of herbs and spices can add excitement and creativity to meals while supporting a balanced and healthful lifestyle.

By embracing the healing power of herbs and spices, individuals can cultivate a deeper connection with nature and harness the potential of these ancient remedies to promote health and vitality. Through mindful selection and preparation, the path to wellness becomes both flavorful and enriching, offering a journey of discovery and nourishment for the body and soul.

The Importance of Omega-3 Fatty Acids

Omega-3 fatty acids are essential nutrients that play a critical role in maintaining health and preventing disease. These polyunsaturated fats, found in abundance in certain fish, seeds, and nuts, are integral to the functioning of every cell in the body. Despite their importance, omega-3s are not produced by the body and must be obtained through diet or supplements, making their inclusion in daily nutrition a priority.

The three main types of omega-3 fatty acids are alpha-linolenic acid (ALA), eicosapentaenoic acid (EPA), and docosahexaenoic acid (DHA). ALA is primarily found in plant sources such as flaxseeds, chia seeds, and walnuts, while EPA and DHA are abundant in marine sources like salmon, mackerel, and sardines. Each type of omega-3 offers unique benefits that contribute to overall health.

One of the most well-documented benefits of omega-3 fatty acids is their positive impact on cardiovascular health. These fats help reduce triglyceride levels, lower blood pressure, and decrease the risk of heart disease. By reducing inflammation and preventing the formation of arterial plaques, omega-3s support healthy blood vessels and promote efficient circulation. Incorporating fatty fish into meals a couple of times a week can significantly enhance heart health and reduce the risk of cardiovascular events.

Omega-3 fatty acids also play a vital role in brain health, influencing cognitive function and emotional well-being. DHA, in particular, is a major structural component of the brain and retina. Adequate levels of DHA are crucial for brain development in infants and children and for maintaining cognitive function in adults. Studies have shown that omega-3s can help improve symptoms of depression and anxiety, potentially due to their anti-inflammatory properties and ability to regulate neurotransmitters. Including omega-3-rich foods in the diet can support mental health and enhance cognitive performance.

The anti-inflammatory properties of omega-3 fatty acids make them valuable for individuals suffering from inflammatory conditions such as arthritis. By reducing inflammation, omega-3s can alleviate joint pain and stiffness, improving mobility and quality of life. Regular consumption of omega-3-rich foods or supplements can provide relief for those with rheumatoid arthritis and other inflammatory disorders.

Omega-3s are also known to support eye health. DHA is a key component of the retina, and adequate intake of omega-3s can help prevent age-related macular degeneration, a leading cause of vision loss. Ensuring a sufficient intake of these fatty acids can protect eye health and maintain clear vision as one ages.

Pregnant and breastfeeding women have increased nutritional needs, and omega-3 fatty acids are particularly important during this time. DHA supports the development of the fetal brain and eyes, and adequate intake during pregnancy can enhance cognitive and visual development in infants. Consuming omega-3-rich foods or supplements during pregnancy and lactation can provide essential nutrients for both mother and child.

For those seeking to incorporate more omega-3s into their diet, a variety of delicious and nutritious options are available. Fatty fish such as salmon, sardines, and trout are excellent sources of EPA and DHA. These can be grilled, baked, or poached and paired with fresh vegetables for a balanced meal. Plant-based sources of ALA, like flaxseeds, chia seeds, and walnuts, can be added to smoothies, oatmeal, salads, or baked goods for an omega-3 boost.

Supplements, such as fish oil or algae oil capsules, are convenient options for those who may not consume enough omega-3-rich foods. When choosing supplements, it's important to select high-quality products that are free from contaminants and provide adequate levels of EPA and DHA. Consulting with a healthcare professional can help determine the appropriate dosage and ensure that supplements fit into a balanced diet.

Balancing omega-3 and omega-6 fatty acids is essential for optimal health. While both are important, the modern diet often provides an excess of omega-6s, found in vegetable oils and processed foods. This imbalance can lead to increased inflammation and health issues. By consciously increasing omega-3 intake and reducing omega-6 consumption, individuals can promote a healthier balance and reduce the risk of chronic diseases.

Incorporating omega-3-rich foods into daily meals requires creativity and a willingness to experiment with different flavors and textures. A breakfast smoothie with chia seeds and spinach, a lunch salad topped with grilled salmon, or a dinner featuring roasted walnuts and vegetables can provide a delicious and nutritious way to boost omega-3 intake. Snacking on walnuts or enjoying a piece of smoked mackerel can further enhance dietary variety and nutrition.

Understanding the importance of omega-3 fatty acids empowers individuals to make informed dietary choices that support overall health and well-being. By embracing the nutritional power of these essential fats, individuals can protect their hearts, enhance brain function, and promote a balanced and fulfilling lifestyle. Through mindful selection and preparation of omega-3-rich foods, the journey to optimal health becomes both enjoyable and rewarding.

Incorporating Healing Foods into Every Meal

Incorporating healing foods into every meal is not just a trend; it is a meaningful approach to nourishing the body and supporting overall health. By thoughtfully selecting ingredients that provide essential nutrients, antioxidants, and other beneficial compounds, individuals can transform their daily meals into powerful tools for well-being. This journey involves creativity, awareness, and a willingness to explore the vast array of healing foods available.

Breakfast is often heralded as the most important meal of the day, setting the tone for energy levels and mood. Starting the day with nutrient-dense foods can provide the necessary fuel for optimal performance and focus. Consider beginning the morning with a bowl of oatmeal topped with fresh berries, a sprinkle of chia seeds, and a dollop of almond butter. The oats provide complex carbohydrates for sustained energy, while the berries offer antioxidants to fight oxidative stress. Chia seeds add omega-3 fatty acids and fiber, promoting heart health and digestion. Almond butter contributes healthy fats and protein, keeping hunger at bay and supporting brain function.

For those who prefer a savory start, an avocado toast topped with a poached egg and a sprinkle of turmeric can be a delightful option. The creamy avocado is rich in monounsaturated fats, which support heart health, while the egg provides high-quality protein and essential nutrients like choline. Turmeric, with its active compound curcumin, adds anti-inflammatory benefits and a burst of color to the plate. A side of sautéed spinach or kale can enhance the meal with additional vitamins and minerals, setting a nourishing foundation for the day.

Lunch is an opportunity to replenish energy and maintain focus throughout the afternoon. A hearty salad featuring a variety of colorful vegetables, lean proteins, and healing herbs can provide a balanced and satisfying meal. Mixed greens such as spinach, arugula, and romaine offer a base rich in vitamins and antioxidants. Top the greens with cherry tomatoes, shredded carrots, and bell peppers for a burst of color and flavor. Grilled chicken, quinoa, or chickpeas can provide protein, while a handful of nuts or seeds adds healthy fats and crunch.

To elevate the salad's healing potential, incorporate herbs like basil, cilantro, or parsley, which offer detoxifying properties and enhance flavor. Dress the salad with a homemade vinaigrette made from olive oil, lemon juice, and a touch of Dijon mustard for an anti-inflammatory and heart-healthy dressing. For an added boost, consider adding fermented foods like sauerkraut or kimchi, which introduce probiotics to support gut health and digestion.

Dinner is a time to unwind and enjoy a nourishing meal that supports relaxation and recovery. A balanced dinner can include lean proteins, whole grains, and a variety of vegetables. Consider preparing a baked salmon fillet, seasoned with garlic and dill, served alongside quinoa and roasted Brussels sprouts. Salmon is an excellent source of omega-3 fatty acids, which support heart and brain health, while quinoa provides a complete protein and essential amino acids. Brussels sprouts, part of the cruciferous vegetable family, are rich in fiber and antioxidants, promoting detoxification and reducing inflammation.

For a plant-based option, a vegetable stir-fry with tofu, broccoli, and bell peppers can offer a satisfying and nutrient-dense meal. Tofu provides a plant-based protein source and is rich in calcium and iron. Broccoli, another cruciferous vegetable, supports detoxification and hormonal balance. Bell peppers add color, sweetness, and vitamin C, enhancing the immune system. A drizzle of tamari or a sprinkle of sesame seeds can elevate the dish with additional flavor and nutrients.

Snacks and beverages also present opportunities to incorporate healing foods. A mid-morning or afternoon snack can include a handful of mixed nuts, providing healthy fats and protein to sustain energy levels. Fresh fruit, such as an apple or a pear, paired with a slice of cheese or a spoonful of nut butter, offers fiber and natural sweetness. For a refreshing beverage, consider a green smoothie made with spinach, banana, almond milk, and a scoop of spirulina. This nutrient-packed drink delivers vitamins, minerals, and antioxidants to support overall health.

Herbal teas can also play a role in incorporating healing foods throughout the day. A cup of chamomile tea can promote relaxation and reduce stress, while peppermint tea aids digestion and provides a refreshing break. Ginger tea, with its warming and spicy notes, can soothe the stomach and support the immune system. Sipping on herbal teas can offer a moment of mindfulness and self-care, enhancing well-being and tranquility.

Creatively incorporating healing foods into every meal involves a willingness to experiment with new ingredients and flavors. Exploring different cuisines and cooking methods can inspire a diverse and balanced diet. For example, Mediterranean dishes often feature olive oil, tomatoes, and herbs, while Asian cuisines highlight the use of ginger, garlic, and fermented foods. Drawing inspiration from various culinary traditions can enrich meals and provide a broad spectrum of nutrients.

Planning and preparation are key to successfully incorporating healing foods into daily life. Keeping a well-stocked pantry with staples such as whole grains, nuts, seeds, and herbs can make meal preparation more efficient and enjoyable. Fresh produce, lean proteins, and fermented foods can be incorporated into weekly meal plans, ensuring a variety of flavors and nutrients. Batch cooking and meal prepping can save time and provide convenient options for busy days.

By embracing the diversity and abundance of healing foods, individuals can cultivate a vibrant and healthful lifestyle. Each meal becomes an opportunity to nourish the body, support wellness, and enjoy the pleasure of delicious and wholesome food. Through mindful selection and preparation, the journey to optimal health becomes an engaging and rewarding experience, fostering a deeper connection to the nourishing power of nature.

Chapter 3: Nutritional Strategies for Common Health Issues

Managing Inflammation with Diet

Inflammation is the body's natural response to injury or illness, acting as a defense mechanism to initiate healing. However, when inflammation becomes chronic, it can contribute to various health problems, including arthritis, cardiovascular disease, and autoimmune disorders. Managing inflammation through diet is a proactive approach to support the body's healing processes and prevent long-term damage. By incorporating anti-inflammatory foods and minimizing pro-inflammatory triggers, individuals can cultivate a diet that promotes balance and wellness.

Central to an anti-inflammatory diet is the emphasis on whole, unprocessed foods rich in nutrients and antioxidants. These foods help neutralize free radicals and reduce oxidative stress, which can exacerbate inflammation. Colorful fruits and vegetables are abundant in antioxidants and phytochemicals that support the immune system and combat inflammation. Including a variety of produce such as berries, leafy greens, and cruciferous vegetables ensures a diverse intake of beneficial compounds.

Berries, including strawberries, blueberries, and raspberries, are particularly high in antioxidants like anthocyanins, which have been shown to reduce inflammation and protect against chronic diseases. Consuming a handful of berries as a snack or adding them to breakfast cereals, yogurt, or smoothies can provide a sweet and nutritious boost. Leafy greens such as spinach, kale, and Swiss chard are rich in vitamins A, C, and K, as well as minerals like magnesium and iron, which support overall health and reduce inflammation.

Cruciferous vegetables, including broccoli, cauliflower, and Brussels sprouts, contain sulforaphane, a compound known for its anti-inflammatory properties. Roasting these vegetables or adding them to stir-fries and salads can enhance meals with flavor and nutrition. Incorporating a wide range of vegetables into the diet not only adds variety but also provides an array of nutrients that work synergistically to combat inflammation.

Healthy fats play a crucial role in managing inflammation. Omega-3 fatty acids, found in fatty fish like salmon, mackerel, and sardines, are known for their anti-inflammatory effects. These fats help reduce the production of inflammatory molecules and support heart and brain health. Including fish in the diet a few times a week can provide a significant source of omega-3s. For those following a plant-based diet, flaxseeds, chia seeds, and walnuts are excellent sources of alpha-linolenic acid (ALA), a type of omega-3 fatty acid. Adding these seeds to smoothies, oatmeal, or salads can boost their nutritional value.

Monounsaturated fats, such as those found in olive oil, avocados, and nuts, also offer anti-inflammatory benefits. Olive oil, a staple of the Mediterranean diet, contains oleocanthal, a compound with effects similar to non-steroidal anti-inflammatory drugs (NSAIDs). Drizzling olive oil over salads, using it in cooking, or dipping bread into it can enhance both flavor and health. Avocados, rich in monounsaturated fats, fiber, and potassium, can be sliced onto sandwiches, blended into smoothies, or enjoyed as a creamy topping for meals.

Whole grains are another important component of an anti-inflammatory diet. Unlike refined grains, which can spike blood sugar levels and promote inflammation, whole grains are high in fiber and nutrients. Quinoa, brown rice, oats, and whole wheat products provide sustained energy and support digestive health. Incorporating these grains into meals can help maintain stable blood sugar levels and decrease inflammation.

Herbs and spices are not only flavorful additions to meals but also possess potent anti-inflammatory properties. Turmeric, with its active compound curcumin, is renowned for its ability to fight inflammation and oxidative stress. Adding turmeric to curries, soups, and teas can introduce its benefits into the diet. Ginger, another powerful spice, can reduce inflammation and soothe digestive issues. Fresh ginger can be grated into dishes or steeped in hot water for a comforting tea.

Garlic, rich in sulfur compounds, has been shown to reduce inflammation and bolster the immune system. Incorporating garlic into sauces, dressings, and roasted vegetables can enhance both taste and health benefits. Cinnamon, with its warming flavor, can help regulate blood sugar and reduce inflammation. Sprinkling it onto oatmeal, smoothies, or baked goods offers a delicious way to enjoy its benefits.

While focusing on anti-inflammatory foods, it's equally important to minimize or avoid foods that can exacerbate inflammation. Processed foods, high in refined sugars and trans fats, can trigger inflammatory responses and increase the risk of chronic diseases. Limiting the consumption of sugary snacks, sodas, and fried foods can support a balanced and healthful diet. Reducing the intake of red and processed meats, which contain inflammatory compounds, can also be beneficial.

Alcohol, when consumed in excess, can contribute to inflammation and liver damage. Moderation is key, and choosing antioxidant-rich options like red wine, in small amounts, may offer some protective benefits. It's essential to be mindful of individual triggers and sensitivities, as certain foods may cause inflammation in some people but not others. Keeping a food diary can help identify any patterns or reactions.

Hydration is another critical component of managing inflammation. Drinking plenty of water supports cellular function and helps flush out toxins that can contribute to inflammation. Herbal teas, such as green tea, chamomile, and peppermint, provide hydration and additional anti-inflammatory benefits. Green tea, rich in catechins, has been shown to reduce inflammation and support heart health.

Lifestyle factors, such as stress management and regular physical activity, also play a role in managing inflammation. Chronic stress can increase inflammatory markers, so incorporating relaxation techniques like meditation, yoga, or deep breathing exercises can be beneficial. Regular exercise, tailored to individual fitness levels, can reduce inflammation and support overall health.

Creating an anti-inflammatory diet involves gradual changes and mindful choices. Planning meals around whole foods, experimenting with new recipes, and exploring different cuisines can make the process enjoyable and sustainable. By prioritizing foods that nourish and heal the body, individuals can support their health and reduce the risk of inflammation-related conditions. Through conscious eating and lifestyle choices, the path to wellness becomes both achievable and fulfilling, fostering a sense of vitality and balance.

Supporting Heart Health Through Nutrition

Heart health is a cornerstone of overall well-being, and nutrition plays an integral role in maintaining a strong and resilient cardiovascular system. By understanding the relationship between diet and heart health, individuals can make informed choices that support their hearts and reduce the risk of heart disease. This journey involves embracing a variety of heart-friendly foods, recognizing potential dietary pitfalls, and creating a balanced approach to eating that nurtures the heart.

Central to supporting heart health is the inclusion of a diverse range of fruits and vegetables in the diet. These nutrient-dense foods are rich in vitamins, minerals, and antioxidants that help protect the heart and reduce the risk of cardiovascular diseases. Leafy greens such as kale, spinach, and collard greens are particularly beneficial, providing high levels of vitamin K, which supports healthy blood clotting, and nitrates that help lower blood pressure. Incorporating these greens into salads, smoothies, and side dishes can enhance meals with flavor and nutrition.

Berries, including strawberries, blueberries, and blackberries, are another powerful ally for the heart. Rich in antioxidants like anthocyanins, berries help reduce oxidative stress and inflammation, two key contributors to heart disease. Enjoying a bowl of mixed berries as a snack or adding them to breakfast cereals and yogurt can provide a delicious and heart-healthy treat.

Whole grains are an essential component of a heart-healthy diet. Unlike refined grains, which can spike blood sugar levels and contribute to weight gain, whole grains retain their fiber and nutrient content, supporting digestive health and maintaining stable energy levels. Oats, brown rice, quinoa, and whole wheat products offer a steady source of energy and help lower cholesterol levels. Incorporating whole grains into daily meals can promote heart health and provide sustained energy throughout the day.

Healthy fats, particularly those found in fish, nuts, and seeds, are vital for cardiovascular support. Omega-3 fatty acids, abundant in fatty fish such as salmon, trout, and sardines, have been shown to reduce triglyceride levels, lower blood pressure, and decrease the risk of heart disease. Including these fish in the diet at least twice a week can provide a significant boost to heart health. For those following a plant-based diet, chia seeds, flaxseeds, and walnuts offer a rich source of omega-3s, which can be added to smoothies, cereals, and salads.

Monounsaturated fats, present in olive oil, avocados, and nuts, also contribute to heart health by reducing bad cholesterol levels and increasing good cholesterol levels. Olive oil, a staple of the Mediterranean diet, is known for its cardiovascular benefits and can be used in cooking, dressings, and as a flavorful dip. Avocados, with their creamy texture and heart-healthy fats, can be enjoyed on toast, in salads, or blended into smoothies for a satisfying and nutritious addition to meals.

In addition to healthy fats, lean proteins play a crucial role in supporting heart health. Skinless poultry, beans, lentils, and tofu provide high-quality protein without the saturated fat found in red and processed meats. These protein sources can be incorporated into a variety of dishes, from hearty soups and stews to salads and stir-fries, offering versatility and nutrition.

Limiting sodium intake is another important aspect of heart health. High sodium levels can contribute to high blood pressure, a significant risk factor for heart disease. Choosing fresh, whole foods over processed and packaged options can help reduce sodium consumption. When seasoning dishes, herbs and spices can be used to enhance flavor without the need for added salt. Experimenting with flavors like garlic, ginger, and rosemary can elevate meals while supporting heart health.

Reducing sugar intake is equally important, as excessive sugar consumption can lead to weight gain, increased triglyceride levels, and a higher risk of heart disease. Opting for natural sweeteners like honey or maple syrup in moderation, and choosing whole fruits over sugary snacks, can help manage sugar intake while satisfying sweet cravings.

Hydration plays a supportive role in maintaining heart health. Water is essential for overall bodily function and helps maintain proper circulation and fluid balance. Herbal teas, such as hibiscus or green tea, offer hydration with additional cardiovascular benefits. Hibiscus tea has been shown to lower blood pressure, while green tea provides antioxidants that support heart health.

Mindful eating and portion control contribute to heart health by preventing overeating and promoting a balanced diet. Paying attention to hunger cues, savoring each bite, and focusing on the sensory experience of eating can enhance satisfaction and prevent overconsumption. Eating slowly and mindfully can also improve digestion and help individuals make healthier choices.

Incorporating a variety of heart-healthy foods into daily meals requires planning and creativity. Keeping a well-stocked pantry with staples like whole grains, nuts, seeds, and olive oil can simplify meal preparation. Fresh fruits and vegetables can be incorporated into weekly meal plans, ensuring a colorful and nutrient-rich diet. Batch cooking and meal prepping can provide convenient options for busy days, supporting consistent heart-healthy eating habits.

Understanding the impact of nutrition on heart health empowers individuals to make choices that support their well-being and longevity. By embracing a diet rich in fruits, vegetables, whole grains, healthy fats, and lean proteins, individuals can nurture their hearts and reduce the risk of cardiovascular diseases. Through mindful eating and thoughtful preparation, the journey to heart health becomes both enjoyable and fulfilling, fostering a sense of vitality and resilience.

Foods for Optimal Brain Function

The human brain, a marvel of complexity, relies heavily on the nutrients it receives to function at its peak. Just as a high-performance engine requires premium fuel, the brain thrives on specific foods that support cognitive abilities, memory, focus, and overall mental health. Understanding which foods bolster brain function can empower individuals to make dietary choices that enhance their cognitive prowess and promote long-term neurological health.

Among the most impactful foods for brain health are those rich in omega-3 fatty acids. These essential fats, particularly docosahexaenoic acid (DHA) and eicosapentaenoic acid (EPA), are critical for maintaining the structure and function of brain cells. Fatty fish such as salmon, mackerel, and sardines are excellent sources of these omega-3s. Regular consumption of these fish can improve memory and reduce the risk of cognitive decline. For vegetarians or those with fish allergies, flaxseeds, chia seeds, and walnuts offer plant-based alternatives rich in alpha-linolenic acid (ALA), which the body can partially convert into DHA and EPA.

Antioxidant-rich foods are another cornerstone of a brain-boosting diet. Berries, such as blueberries, strawberries, and blackberries, are packed with antioxidants, particularly flavonoids, which have been shown to enhance communication between brain cells, improve memory, and reduce inflammation. Incorporating a variety of berries into daily meals, whether as a topping for yogurt or blended into smoothies, provides a delicious way to support cognitive function.

Leafy greens like spinach, kale, and Swiss chard are loaded with brain-healthy nutrients, including vitamins K, A, and E, as well as folate and iron. These nutrients are essential for neuroprotection and cognitive function. Regular consumption of leafy greens can slow cognitive decline and preserve brain health. Adding them to salads, smoothies, or side dishes can easily increase their presence in the diet.

Nuts and seeds, beyond their omega-3 content, provide a wealth of nutrients that support brain health. Almonds, hazelnuts, and sunflower seeds are rich in vitamin E, which has been linked to reduced cognitive decline as people age. A handful of mixed nuts or seeds can be a convenient snack that provides both satiety and brain benefits.

Whole grains are vital for providing the brain with a steady supply of energy. Unlike refined grains, which can cause spikes in blood sugar levels, whole grains release glucose slowly into the bloodstream, maintaining consistent energy levels throughout the day. Oats, brown rice, and quinoa are excellent choices that can be incorporated into breakfasts, lunches, and dinners to support sustained cognitive function.

Dark chocolate, in moderation, is a delightful treat that offers brain benefits due to its high concentration of flavonoids, caffeine, and antioxidants. These compounds can enhance memory, improve mood, and boost overall brain function. Choosing high-quality dark chocolate with at least 70% cocoa content and enjoying small portions can satisfy sweet cravings while supporting mental acuity.

Avocados, known for their creamy texture, are rich in healthy fats and potassium, both of which support healthy blood flow and lower blood pressure. Proper circulation is crucial for optimal brain function, as it ensures that the brain receives an adequate supply of oxygen and nutrients. Adding avocado to salads, sandwiches, or smoothies can enhance both the flavor and nutritional profile of meals.

Broccoli, a cruciferous vegetable, is an excellent source of antioxidants and vitamin K, which is vital for forming sphingolipids, a type of fat densely packed into brain cells. Consuming broccoli regularly can support cognitive function and protect against neurological disorders. Roasting or steaming broccoli as a side dish, or incorporating it into stir-fries, can make this brain-friendly vegetable a regular part of the diet.

Turmeric, a golden spice renowned for its anti-inflammatory properties, contains curcumin, which can cross the blood-brain barrier and benefit the brain. Curcumin may help improve memory and stimulate the production of brain-derived neurotrophic factor (BDNF), a growth hormone that encourages the formation of new neural connections. Incorporating turmeric into curries, soups, or golden milk can introduce its cognitive benefits into the diet.

Hydration is often overlooked but is vital for maintaining concentration and alertness. The brain is composed of about 75% water, and even mild dehydration can impair cognitive performance. Drinking plenty of water throughout the day, alongside herbal teas such as green tea, which provides additional antioxidants and caffeine, can support sustained mental function.

Lifestyle factors also contribute to optimal brain function. Regular physical activity, quality sleep, and stress management are essential for maintaining cognitive health. Exercise increases blood flow to the brain, enhancing its function and encouraging the release of beneficial neurotransmitters. Adequate sleep is crucial for memory consolidation and clearing toxins from the brain. Stress management techniques, such as mindfulness meditation and deep breathing exercises, can reduce cortisol levels and promote mental clarity.

Creating a brain-boosting diet involves thoughtful planning and a willingness to experiment with new foods and recipes. Stocking the pantry with nutrient-dense staples like whole grains, nuts, seeds, and spices can simplify meal preparation and ensure a steady supply of brain-supportive ingredients. Fresh produce, including berries, leafy greens, and avocados, can be incorporated into weekly meal plans, providing a colorful and nutrient-rich diet.

Understanding the profound impact of nutrition on brain function empowers individuals to make dietary choices that enhance cognitive health and support long-term mental well-being. By incorporating a variety of brain-friendly foods into daily meals, individuals can nurture their cognitive abilities and reduce the risk of neurological decline. Through mindful eating and lifestyle choices, the journey to optimal brain health becomes both rewarding and sustainable, fostering a sense of vitality and mental clarity.

Strengthening Immunity with Food

The immune system, a complex network of cells, tissues, and organs, serves as the body's primary defense against infections and diseases. While genetics and lifestyle factors play a role in immune health, nutrition is a powerful, modifiable factor that can significantly enhance the body's ability to ward off illness. By incorporating specific foods known to bolster immune function, individuals can fortify their defenses and promote resilience in the face of health challenges.

A diet rich in fruits and vegetables is foundational to supporting immunity. These vibrant foods provide a wealth of essential vitamins, minerals, and antioxidants that help protect and repair cells. Citrus fruits, such as oranges, grapefruits, lemons, and limes, are celebrated for their high vitamin C content. This vitamin is crucial for the production of white blood cells, which are key players in immune response. Enjoying a glass of freshly squeezed orange juice or adding lemon to meals can provide a refreshing dose of this immune-supportive nutrient.

Beyond citrus, other fruits like kiwi, strawberries, and papaya also offer ample vitamin C along with additional nutrients. Kiwi, for instance, is rich in vitamin E and potassium, contributing to overall health. Incorporating a variety of these fruits into the diet can ensure a comprehensive intake of immune-boosting compounds.

Vegetables, particularly those that are dark and leafy, are packed with vitamins and minerals essential for immune function. Spinach, kale, and Swiss chard are rich in vitamin A, iron, and folate, which play roles in maintaining the integrity of mucosal barriers and supporting immune cell activity. These leafy greens can be easily added to salads, soups, or smoothies, enhancing meals with their nutritional value.

Cruciferous vegetables like broccoli, Brussels sprouts, and cauliflower contain sulforaphane, a compound that has been shown to boost the production of antioxidant enzymes in the body. These enzymes help neutralize free radicals and reduce oxidative stress, both of which can weaken the immune system. Roasting or steaming these vegetables can make them a tasty and nutritious addition to the diet.

Garlic, a kitchen staple known for its pungent flavor, is a powerful ally in immune support. It contains allicin, a sulfur-containing compound with antiviral and antibacterial properties. Regular consumption of garlic can enhance immune response and reduce the severity of colds and other infections. Adding crushed or chopped garlic to sauces, dressings, and marinades can provide both flavor and health benefits.

Ginger, another potent spice, has anti-inflammatory and antioxidant properties that can support immune health. It can help reduce inflammation and soothe symptoms of colds and sore throats. Fresh ginger can be grated into teas, stir-fries, or smoothies, offering a warming and therapeutic component to meals.

Fermented foods play a unique role in strengthening immunity by promoting gut health. A significant portion of the immune system resides in the gut, where beneficial bacteria help regulate immune responses. Foods like yogurt, kefir, sauerkraut, kimchi, and miso are rich in probiotics, which support a healthy balance of gut flora. Incorporating these foods into the diet can enhance digestive health and improve the body's ability to fend off pathogens.

Adequate protein intake is essential for the production of immune cells and antibodies. Lean meats, poultry, fish, eggs, and legumes provide high-quality protein that supports immune function. Zinc, a mineral found in abundance in shellfish, nuts, seeds, and legumes, is also crucial for immune health. It supports the development and communication of immune cells and helps the body heal wounds. Including these foods in meals can ensure sufficient protein and zinc intake.

Hydration is another important factor in maintaining a robust immune system. Water helps transport nutrients to cells and remove waste products, supporting overall bodily function. Herbal teas, such as echinacea, elderberry, and green tea, offer hydration with additional immune-supportive benefits. Echinacea and elderberry have been traditionally used to reduce the duration and severity of colds, while green tea provides antioxidants that support immune health.

Vitamin D, known as the "sunshine vitamin," is essential for immune regulation. While the body can produce vitamin D through sun exposure, dietary sources are also important, especially in regions with limited sunlight. Fatty fish like salmon and mackerel, fortified dairy products, and egg yolks are good sources of vitamin D. Including these foods in the diet can help maintain adequate vitamin D levels, supporting immune resilience.

Nuts and seeds, especially almonds and sunflower seeds, are rich in vitamin E, an antioxidant that enhances immune function. A handful of these seeds can be a convenient snack that provides both energy and immune support.

Incorporating a variety of these immune-boosting foods into daily meals requires planning and creativity. Keeping a well-stocked pantry with essentials like garlic, ginger, nuts, and seeds can simplify meal preparation. Fresh fruits and vegetables can be planned into weekly meals, ensuring a colorful and nutrient-rich diet. Fermented foods and lean protein sources can be included in recipes, providing balance and diversity.

Understanding the impact of nutrition on immune health empowers individuals to make choices that support their well-being and resilience. By embracing a diet rich in fruits, vegetables, lean proteins, and fermented foods, individuals can nurture their immune systems and enhance their body's natural defenses. Through mindful eating and thoughtful preparation, the journey to optimal immune health becomes both achievable and rewarding, fostering a sense of vitality and well-being.

Balancing Blood Sugar and Metabolism

Balancing blood sugar and optimizing metabolism are essential for maintaining energy levels, supporting weight management, and reducing the risk of chronic diseases such as diabetes. Understanding the relationship between diet, blood sugar, and metabolism allows individuals to make informed choices that promote stable glucose levels and efficient metabolic function.

The body's ability to regulate blood sugar hinges on the consumption of carbohydrates, which are broken down into glucose in the bloodstream. Choosing complex carbohydrates over simple ones is crucial for maintaining stable blood sugar levels. Unlike simple carbohydrates, which can cause rapid spikes and crashes in blood sugar, complex carbohydrates are digested more slowly, providing a steady release of glucose. Whole grains like quinoa, oats, and brown rice are excellent sources of complex carbohydrates. Incorporating these grains into meals can provide sustained energy and prevent the rollercoaster effect of blood sugar fluctuations.

Fiber plays a pivotal role in balancing blood sugar. Foods rich in fiber slow down the absorption of sugar into the bloodstream, preventing sharp spikes. Fruits, vegetables, legumes, and whole grains are abundant in fiber, making them essential components of a balanced diet. For example, pairing fiber-rich beans with meals not only enhances satiety but also stabilizes blood sugar levels. Including a variety of colorful vegetables and legumes in daily meals can ensure adequate fiber intake.

Protein is another key player in regulating blood sugar and metabolism. By slowing digestion and reducing the glycemic response of meals, protein helps maintain stable glucose levels. Lean protein sources such as chicken, turkey, fish, tofu, and legumes can be incorporated into a variety of dishes, from salads to stir-fries, providing versatility and nutrition. For instance, adding grilled chicken to a salad or tofu to a vegetable stir-fry can enhance both flavor and blood sugar control.

Healthy fats are vital for sustaining energy and supporting metabolic health. Unlike refined carbohydrates, fats do not cause spikes in blood sugar levels. Avocados, nuts, seeds, and olive oil are excellent sources of healthy fats that can be included in meals to promote satiety and balanced energy. A handful of almonds as a snack or a drizzle of olive oil over roasted vegetables can contribute to a nutritious and satisfying diet.

Understanding the glycemic index (GI) of foods can guide choices that support balanced blood sugar levels. The GI measures how quickly a food raises blood sugar levels. Foods with a low GI, such as lentils, chickpeas, and non-starchy vegetables, release glucose slowly and steadily, making them ideal for maintaining stable blood sugar. Incorporating low-GI foods into meals can help manage cravings and sustain energy throughout the day.

Portion control is a crucial aspect of balancing blood sugar and metabolism. Even healthy foods can lead to imbalances if consumed in excessive amounts. Mindful eating practices, such as paying attention to hunger cues and savoring each bite, can enhance satisfaction and prevent overeating. Eating slowly and engaging the senses can lead to better portion control and improved digestion.

Meal timing and frequency also play roles in blood sugar regulation. Eating smaller, balanced meals at regular intervals can prevent extreme fluctuations in blood sugar levels. Skipping meals or waiting too long between meals can lead to blood sugar crashes and increased cravings. Planning for regular meals and snacks that include a balance of carbohydrates, protein, and healthy fats can support stable blood sugar and metabolic function.

Hydration is often overlooked but is essential for metabolic health. Water is involved in numerous metabolic processes, and even mild dehydration can slow metabolism. Drinking adequate water throughout the day supports overall health and ensures efficient metabolic function. Herbal teas, such as peppermint or chamomile, offer hydration with additional soothing benefits.

Physical activity complements dietary efforts to balance blood sugar and enhance metabolism. Regular exercise increases insulin sensitivity, allowing cells to use glucose more effectively. Incorporating both aerobic and strength-training exercises into a weekly routine can improve metabolic health and support weight management. Activities like walking, cycling, or yoga can be enjoyable ways to stay active and promote blood sugar balance.

Stress management is another important component of blood sugar regulation. Chronic stress can elevate cortisol levels, leading to increased blood sugar and insulin resistance. Incorporating relaxation techniques such as meditation, deep breathing exercises, or mindfulness practices can reduce stress and support metabolic health. Taking time for self-care and stress-relief activities can enhance overall well-being and facilitate balanced blood sugar levels.

Creating a diet that supports balanced blood sugar and metabolism involves thoughtful planning and preparation. Keeping a well-stocked pantry with whole grains, lean proteins, and healthy fats can simplify meal preparation and ensure access to nutritious ingredients. Fresh fruits and vegetables can be incorporated into weekly meal plans, providing a colorful and nutrient-rich diet. Batch cooking and meal prepping can offer convenient options for busy days, supporting consistent healthy eating habits.

Understanding the impact of nutrition on blood sugar and metabolism empowers individuals to make choices that enhance their well-being and vitality. By embracing a diet rich in fiber, complex carbohydrates, lean proteins, and healthy fats, individuals can nurture their metabolic health and maintain stable blood sugar levels. Through mindful eating and lifestyle practices, the journey to balanced blood sugar and optimized metabolism becomes both achievable and rewarding, fostering a sense of energy and resilience.

Chapter 4: Creating a Healing Kitchen

Stocking Your Pantry with Nutritional Powerhouses

In the world of nutrition, a well-stocked pantry is akin to a painter's palette, brimming with the ingredients needed to craft vibrant, healthful meals. For beginners venturing into the realm of nutritious cooking, understanding which foods serve as nutritional powerhouses can simplify meal preparation and ensure a balanced diet. By strategically filling the pantry with essential ingredients, one can create a foundation for countless delicious and nourishing dishes.

Whole grains are fundamental components of a nutritious pantry. Unlike refined grains, whole grains retain their bran and germ, offering a rich source of fiber, vitamins, and minerals. Brown rice, quinoa, oats, and farro are versatile staples that can be incorporated into breakfast, lunch, or dinner. These grains provide sustained energy and support digestive health. Imagine waking up to a warm bowl of oatmeal topped with fresh berries and nuts or enjoying a hearty quinoa salad for lunch, brimming with colorful vegetables and a zesty dressing.

Legumes, including beans, lentils, and chickpeas, are nutritional powerhouses packed with protein, fiber, and essential nutrients. They are not only budget-friendly but also incredibly versatile. From soups and stews to salads and dips, legumes can transform a simple dish into a satisfying meal. Picture a comforting bowl of lentil soup on a chilly evening or a vibrant chickpea salad tossed with lemon and herbs for a refreshing summer lunch.

Nuts and seeds are small but mighty additions to the pantry, offering healthy fats, protein, and an array of vitamins and minerals. Almonds, walnuts, chia seeds, and flaxseeds are excellent choices that can enhance both sweet and savory dishes. A handful of almonds can serve as a quick snack, while chia seeds soaked overnight in almond milk create a delicious pudding perfect for breakfast. Incorporating nuts and seeds into meals not only boosts nutrition but also adds delightful textures and flavors.

Herbs and spices are the unsung heroes of any pantry, transforming ordinary ingredients into extraordinary meals. Beyond their ability to enhance flavor, many herbs and spices offer health benefits. Turmeric, known for its anti-inflammatory properties, can be added to curries or golden milk. Cinnamon, which helps regulate blood sugar, can be sprinkled over oatmeal or mixed into smoothies. A well-curated spice rack invites culinary creativity and exploration, allowing you to travel the world through your taste buds without leaving the kitchen.

Canned and jarred goods provide convenience without sacrificing nutrition. Canned tomatoes, coconut milk, and vegetable broth are versatile ingredients that form the base of numerous recipes. When selecting canned goods, opt for those with no added sugars or preservatives to ensure you're getting the purest form of the ingredient. Imagine whipping up a quick tomato sauce for pasta or a creamy coconut curry in minutes with these pantry staples.

Healthy oils are essential for cooking and dressing dishes. Olive oil, renowned for its monounsaturated fats and heart-healthy properties, is a staple for Mediterranean-inspired meals. Coconut oil, with its subtle sweetness, is perfect for baking or sautéing. These oils not only enhance the flavor of dishes but also contribute to overall health. Drizzling olive oil over roasted vegetables or using coconut oil in baking can elevate both taste and nutrition.

Vinegars and condiments add depth and complexity to dishes. Balsamic vinegar, apple cider vinegar, and soy sauce are versatile pantry items that can be used to create marinades, dressings, and sauces. A splash of balsamic vinegar can brighten a salad, while a dash of soy sauce can add umami to stir-fries. These condiments allow for experimentation and customization, making each meal unique.

Dried fruits, such as apricots, raisins, and dates, offer natural sweetness and can be used in both savory and sweet dishes. They are rich in fiber and antioxidants, making them a nutritious addition to the pantry. Dates can be blended into smoothies for a natural sweetener, while raisins can be added to salads for a burst of sweetness. These fruits are perfect for snacking or enhancing the flavor and nutrition of meals.

Seafood, whether fresh or canned, provides a rich source of omega-3 fatty acids and protein. Canned tuna or salmon is convenient and can be used in salads, sandwiches, or pasta dishes. Fresh seafood can be stored in the freezer and thawed for a special meal. Incorporating seafood into the diet supports heart health and adds variety to meals.

Frozen fruits and vegetables are practical additions to the pantry, offering nutrition and convenience. Flash-frozen at peak ripeness, they retain their nutrients and can be stored for long periods. Frozen berries can be blended into smoothies or added to yogurt, while frozen vegetables can be tossed into soups or stir-fries. Having these items on hand ensures you always have access to nutritious ingredients, even on the busiest days.

Building a pantry with these nutritional powerhouses provides a solid foundation for healthful eating. By having these ingredients readily available, you can create meals that are both nourishing and satisfying. The pantry becomes a source of inspiration, encouraging culinary creativity and experimentation. It empowers you to make choices that enhance well-being, transforming the act of cooking into a joyful and rewarding experience.

Understanding the impact of a well-stocked pantry on health and well-being allows individuals to take control of their nutrition and culinary journey. By embracing a diverse array of whole grains, legumes, nuts, seeds, herbs, and other nutritional powerhouses, individuals can craft delicious and nourishing meals with ease. Through thoughtful selection and mindful preparation, the pantry becomes a gateway to vibrant health and culinary adventure, fostering a sense of empowerment and joy in the kitchen.

Cooking Techniques that Preserve Nutrients

Cooking is an art that not only satisfies our taste buds but also fuels our bodies with the nutrients we need to thrive. However, the methods we use to prepare food can significantly impact the nutritional value of our meals. Preserving nutrients during cooking is essential for maintaining the health benefits of the ingredients we consume. By understanding and applying specific techniques, we can maximize the nutritional content of our meals while still enjoying delicious flavors.

Steaming is one of the most effective cooking methods for preserving nutrients. By using steam rather than submerging vegetables in water, this method minimizes nutrient loss, particularly water-soluble vitamins like vitamin C and B vitamins. Steaming is ideal for leafy greens, broccoli, and carrots, as it maintains their vibrant color and crisp texture. Imagine the subtle aroma of fresh broccoli as it steams gently, ready to be tossed with a drizzle of olive oil and a sprinkle of sesame seeds for a nutritious side dish.

Sautéing is another technique that can help preserve nutrients, especially when done quickly over moderate heat. Using a small amount of healthy fat, such as olive oil or avocado oil, enhances the absorption of fat-soluble vitamins like A, D, E, and K. Sautéing allows for the caramelization of vegetables, which can enhance their natural sweetness. Picture a medley of bell peppers, onions, and zucchini sizzling in a pan, their colors intensifying as they cook to perfection.

Stir-frying, a staple in Asian cuisine, is a fast and efficient way to cook vegetables and proteins while preserving their nutritional integrity. This high-heat method involves continuously tossing ingredients in a wok or large skillet, ensuring even cooking. The key to successful stir-frying is to cut ingredients into uniform pieces, allowing them to cook quickly and retain their nutrients. A vibrant stir-fry with snap peas, carrots, and tofu, seasoned with ginger and garlic, can be a nutrient-packed meal that delights the senses.

Roasting is a cooking method that can concentrate flavors while retaining nutrients, particularly when it comes to root vegetables like sweet potatoes, beets, and parsnips. By using dry heat, roasting caramelizes the natural sugars in vegetables, enhancing their sweetness and depth of flavor. To retain nutrients, it's important not to overcook the vegetables. A tray of roasted carrots and Brussels sprouts, seasoned with rosemary and thyme, can serve as a hearty and nutritious accompaniment to any meal.

Grilling, often associated with outdoor cooking, can be a healthy way to prepare proteins and vegetables. The high heat of grilling sears the food, locking in moisture and flavor while minimizing nutrient loss. To prevent the formation of harmful compounds, it's crucial to avoid charring food and to marinate meats before grilling. A platter of grilled chicken and vegetable skewers, brushed with a tangy lemon and herb marinade, can provide a nutritious and satisfying meal.

Blanching is a technique often used to preserve the color, texture, and nutrients of vegetables. By briefly boiling vegetables and then plunging them into ice water, blanching halts the cooking process and preserves the vibrant colors and nutrients of the vegetables. Blanched green beans or asparagus can be tossed into salads or served as a crisp and colorful side dish.

Microwaving, though often underestimated, can be an efficient way to cook vegetables while preserving their nutritional content. By using minimal water and shorter cooking times, microwaving reduces nutrient loss. Steaming vegetables in the microwave with a small amount of water in a covered dish can be a quick and convenient way to prepare a nutritious meal. A bowl of steamed broccoli, ready in minutes, can be a perfect addition to any dinner plate.

Poaching is a gentle cooking method that involves simmering food in liquid at low temperatures. This technique is ideal for delicate proteins like fish and eggs, as well as fruits. Poaching helps retain nutrients and moisture, resulting in tender and flavorful dishes. A poached salmon fillet, served with a light dill sauce, can be a nutritious and elegant main course.

Pressure cooking, using devices like an Instant Pot, is a modern technique that cooks food quickly under high pressure, preserving nutrients and flavors. This method is particularly effective for legumes and grains, which require longer cooking times. A hearty pressure-cooked lentil stew, infused with spices and herbs, can be a nutrient-dense meal that warms the soul.

Boiling is a method that can lead to nutrient loss, particularly with water-soluble vitamins. However, by minimizing cooking time and using just enough water to cover the food, nutrient retention can be improved. Using the cooking liquid in soups or sauces can also help reclaim lost nutrients. A pot of boiled potatoes, gently mashed with olive oil and garlic, can serve as a comforting and nutritious side dish.

Sous vide, a technique that involves vacuum-sealing food and cooking it in a water bath at precise temperatures, preserves nutrients by maintaining a consistent, low temperature throughout the cooking process. This method is excellent for proteins and vegetables, ensuring even cooking and enhanced flavor. A sous vide chicken breast, tender and juicy, paired with a vibrant vegetable medley, offers a gourmet dining experience with optimal nutrition.

By employing these cooking techniques, you can retain the essential vitamins, minerals, and antioxidants found in fresh ingredients, maximizing the health benefits of your meals. Understanding the science behind each method allows for informed choices that enhance both flavor and nutrition. With a bit of practice and creativity, you can transform your kitchen into a haven of healthful cooking, where every meal becomes an opportunity to nourish both body and soul.

Meal Planning for Health and Wellness

The journey to health and wellness often begins in the kitchen, where meal planning serves as a powerful tool for achieving nutritional goals and maintaining a balanced lifestyle. For beginners, meal planning can seem daunting, but with a few strategies and a bit of creativity, it becomes an empowering practice that saves time, reduces stress, and ensures a diet rich in variety and nutrients.

Meal planning starts with setting realistic and personalized goals. Understanding your nutritional needs, dietary preferences, and lifestyle demands is crucial for creating a plan that aligns with your health objectives. Whether the aim is weight management, energy enhancement, or overall wellness, having clear goals provides direction and motivation. Consider the story of Emily, a busy professional who, after identifying her need for more energy and improved digestion, focused on incorporating whole foods and balanced meals into her weekly plan.

Creating a weekly meal plan involves considering both macro and micronutrients. A balanced plan includes a variety of proteins, carbohydrates, and healthy fats, as well as vitamins and minerals from fruits and vegetables. Incorporating diverse food groups ensures that meals are nutritionally complete and satisfying. For instance, a typical day might include a breakfast of oatmeal with fresh fruit and nuts, a lunch of grilled chicken with quinoa and roasted vegetables, and a dinner of salmon with a side of leafy greens.

A crucial aspect of meal planning is selecting recipes that are both nutritious and aligned with personal taste preferences. Exploring new cuisines and cooking methods can add excitement to meal planning while expanding culinary horizons. Experimenting with flavors and textures keeps meals interesting and prevents monotony. Imagine the delight of discovering a new favorite dish like a spicy Thai curry or a comforting Italian minestrone, each packed with nutrients and flavor.

One of the most practical elements of meal planning is creating a detailed grocery list based on the weekly menu. This list ensures that all necessary ingredients are on hand, reducing the temptation for unhealthy choices and minimizing food waste. Organizing the list by categories, such as produce, proteins, and pantry staples, can streamline the shopping process and save time. Picture yourself navigating the aisles with confidence, knowing exactly what you need to create wholesome meals for the week.

Batch cooking and meal prepping are invaluable techniques for those with busy schedules. By dedicating a few hours each week to cooking and preparing meals in advance, you can ensure that nutritious options are always available, even on the busiest days. Preparing large batches of staples like brown rice, lentils, or roasted vegetables provides a foundation for quick and easy meals. Visualize opening your refrigerator to find neatly stacked containers of colorful, ready-to-eat dishes, each one a testament to your planning and effort.

Flexibility is key to successful meal planning. Life is unpredictable, and plans may need to be adjusted due to unexpected events or changes in schedule. Having a few backup meals, such as homemade soups or frozen casseroles, can provide peace of mind and prevent reliance on takeout or fast food. These backup options serve as a safety net, ensuring that your commitment to health and wellness remains intact, even when circumstances shift.

Incorporating seasonal and local produce into meal planning not only enhances the nutritional quality of meals but also supports local farmers and sustainability efforts. Seasonal produce is often fresher, more flavorful, and more affordable. Visiting a local farmers' market can inspire new recipes and introduce you to ingredients you might not have considered. Envision the vibrant colors and fresh aromas of seasonal fruits and vegetables, each one offering a unique blend of nutrients and flavors.

Mindful eating practices complement meal planning by fostering a deeper connection with the food we consume. Taking time to savor each bite, appreciating the textures and flavors, can enhance the dining experience and improve digestion. Mindful eating encourages listening to hunger cues and recognizing satiety, preventing overeating and supporting weight management. Imagine sitting down to a beautifully arranged plate, free from distractions, allowing yourself to fully enjoy the meal you've thoughtfully prepared.

Engaging family or friends in meal planning and preparation can transform it into a social and enjoyable activity. Involving loved ones in the process not only lightens the load but also introduces diverse perspectives and ideas. Cooking together creates opportunities for bonding and learning, as well as sharing the rewards of a homemade meal. Picture the laughter and camaraderie as you chop vegetables alongside a friend or teach a child how to stir a pot of simmering stew.

The digital age offers a plethora of tools and resources to assist with meal planning. Apps and websites dedicated to nutrition and meal planning can provide inspiration, track nutritional intake, and suggest recipes based on dietary preferences. Leveraging technology can simplify the planning process, offering customized solutions that cater to individual needs. Imagine scrolling through a digital recipe box, filled with curated options that excite your palate and align with your health goals.

Reflecting on the outcomes of meal planning is an important step in refining the process. Taking note of what worked well and what could be improved allows for continuous growth and adaptation. Celebrating small victories, such as trying a new vegetable or successfully sticking to the plan for a week, reinforces positive habits and maintains motivation. Picture yourself at the end of the week, reflecting on the delicious and nutritious meals you've enjoyed, feeling a sense of accomplishment and well-being.

By embracing meal planning, individuals take proactive steps toward achieving their health and wellness goals. The act of planning meals with intention and care transforms the daily routine into a purposeful practice that nourishes both body and mind. With a bit of creativity and dedication, meal planning becomes a cornerstone of a healthy lifestyle, offering both structure and freedom, and ultimately leading to a more balanced and fulfilling life.

Adapting Recipes for Therapeutic Benefits

Cooking is more than just a means to satisfy hunger; it can also be a therapeutic process that supports health and wellness. Adapting recipes to enhance their therapeutic benefits allows individuals to address specific health concerns through the food they consume. By making thoughtful substitutions and additions, one can transform everyday dishes into powerful tools for healing and nourishment.

Understanding the nutritional needs associated with particular health conditions is the first step in adapting recipes for therapeutic benefits. For example, someone managing high blood pressure might focus on reducing sodium intake and increasing potassium-rich foods. On the other hand, an individual with diabetes may prioritize controlling carbohydrate intake and choosing low-glycemic index foods. Tailoring recipes to fit these needs ensures meals contribute positively to overall health.

Substituting ingredients is a practical way to enhance the therapeutic value of a dish. Consider a classic lasagna: by swapping traditional pasta for whole-grain or zucchini noodles, the fiber content increases, supporting digestive health. Replacing regular ricotta cheese with a lower-fat or plant-based alternative can reduce saturated fat intake. These simple changes not only make the dish healthier but also align it with specific dietary goals.

Incorporating herbs and spices with known health benefits is another effective strategy. Turmeric, with its anti-inflammatory properties, can be added to soups, stews, or rice dishes. Ginger, known for its digestive and anti-nausea effects, can be grated into smoothies or teas. By using these natural flavor enhancers, meals gain therapeutic qualities without compromising taste.

For individuals looking to boost their immune system, recipes can be adapted by including ingredients rich in vitamins and antioxidants. A simple chicken soup can become an immunity-boosting powerhouse by adding garlic, onion, and kale. These ingredients are known for their immune-supportive properties, and their inclusion makes the dish both comforting and beneficial during cold and flu season.

For those focused on heart health, adapting recipes to include heart-friendly ingredients can be beneficial. Incorporating fatty fish like salmon, rich in omega-3 fatty acids, into meals can support cardiovascular health. A salad topped with walnuts, avocados, and a drizzle of olive oil provides healthy fats that promote heart health. Each of these additions enhances the nutritional profile of the dish while offering therapeutic benefits.

When adapting recipes for weight management, portion control and nutrient density are key. Recipes can be adjusted to include more vegetables, which are low in calories but high in fiber, helping to increase satiety. A stir-fry can be filled with colorful bell peppers, broccoli, and snap peas, creating a filling meal without excess calories. Making vegetables the star of the dish allows for both satisfaction and nourishment.

For those with dietary restrictions or food allergies, recipe adaptation is essential. Ingredients that may trigger allergic reactions, such as nuts, dairy, or gluten, can be replaced with safe alternatives. Almond milk can substitute for cow's milk, while gluten-free flours can replace wheat flours in baking.

These adaptations ensure that individuals can enjoy meals without compromising their health or safety.

Incorporating fermented foods into recipes can support gut health and digestion. Adding sauerkraut to sandwiches or miso to soups introduces beneficial probiotics that promote a healthy gut microbiome. These foods not only enhance flavor but also provide therapeutic benefits that aid digestion and improve overall gut health.

Adapting recipes to support mental well-being is another important consideration. Foods rich in omega-3 fatty acids, such as flaxseeds and chia seeds, are known to support brain health and mood regulation. Incorporating these seeds into oatmeal or smoothies can provide a mental health boost. Additionally, dark chocolate, rich in antioxidants, can be used in desserts for both indulgence and therapeutic benefit.

Hydration is a vital component of wellness, and recipes can be adapted to include hydrating ingredients. Soups, stews, and smoothies can be enriched with water-dense fruits and vegetables like cucumbers, watermelon, and tomatoes. These additions not only improve hydration but also enhance the nutritional content of the meal.

For those seeking to enhance bone health, adapting recipes to include calcium and vitamin D-rich foods is beneficial. Leafy greens like spinach and kale can be added to casseroles or smoothies, providing calcium along with other essential nutrients. Fortified plant milks can be used in place of dairy, ensuring adequate vitamin D intake. These adaptations support bone health and provide important nutrients in a delicious form.

Adapting recipes also involves considering cooking methods that preserve nutrients. Steaming, roasting, and sautéing are techniques that maintain the nutritional value of ingredients while enhancing flavor. By choosing cooking methods that preserve vitamins and minerals, meals become more nourishing and beneficial.

For individuals interested in boosting energy levels, recipes can be adapted to include complex carbohydrates and protein-rich ingredients. A breakfast of whole-grain toast with avocado and poached eggs provides sustained energy throughout the morning. A snack of hummus with whole-grain crackers offers a balanced mix of carbohydrates and protein, supporting energy levels throughout the day.

Adapting recipes for therapeutic benefits is a creative and rewarding process that empowers individuals to take control of their health through the food they consume. By making intentional choices and substitutions, meals can become not only a source of pleasure but also a means of supporting overall health and well-being. Through thoughtful adaptation, the kitchen becomes a place of healing and nourishment, where each dish is crafted with both taste and therapeutic value in mind.

Chapter 5: Integrating Mindful Eating and Nutrition

The Role of Mindfulness in Healing

Mindfulness, a practice rooted in ancient tradition, has gained widespread recognition for its profound impact on mental, emotional, and physical well-being. Its role in healing is multifaceted, offering individuals a pathway to connect with themselves and their surroundings in a more profound and meaningful way. By fostering a state of present-moment awareness, mindfulness allows us to tap into the body's innate capacity for healing, addressing both visible ailments and hidden stresses.

Consider the story of Sarah, a graphic designer who constantly juggled deadlines and personal obligations. The relentless pace left her feeling anxious and overwhelmed, manifesting in physical symptoms such as tension headaches and fatigue. Desperate for relief, she turned to mindfulness, initially skeptical but willing to explore any avenue for peace. Through daily mindfulness practice, she learned to focus on her breath, acknowledging her thoughts without judgment. Over time, the headaches subsided, replaced by a sense of calm and clarity. Sarah's story is a testament to the transformative power of mindfulness in healing not just the body, but the mind and spirit as well.

Mindfulness encourages individuals to become attuned to their body's signals, fostering an awareness that can prevent minor issues from escalating into significant health concerns. By paying attention to physical sensations, emotional cues, and thought patterns, individuals can identify stressors and triggers, allowing for timely intervention. This heightened awareness acts as a preventative measure, promoting overall health and well-being.

The practice of mindfulness involves several techniques, each with unique benefits. Mindful breathing, for instance, serves as a cornerstone of mindfulness practice. By focusing on the rhythm of the breath, one anchors themselves in the present moment, reducing stress and anxiety. This simple yet powerful technique can be practiced anywhere, offering a moment of respite in a hectic day. Imagine sitting quietly, inhaling deeply, and exhaling slowly, feeling the tension melt away with each breath.

Body scan meditation is another effective mindfulness technique that involves mentally scanning the body from head to toe, acknowledging any sensations without judgment. This practice can unveil areas of tension or discomfort, guiding individuals in addressing physical and emotional needs. Picture lying down in a quiet space, closing your eyes, and slowly bringing your awareness to each part of your body, releasing any tension you encounter along the way.

Mindful movement, such as yoga or tai chi, combines physical activity with mindfulness, promoting flexibility, strength, and relaxation. These practices encourage individuals to move with intention, synchronizing breath with movement, and cultivating a deep connection with the body. Visualize flowing through a series of gentle yoga poses, each movement a dance of mindfulness and grace, bringing a sense of balance and harmony.

Incorporating mindfulness into daily activities further enhances its healing potential. Mindful eating, for example, involves savoring each bite, paying attention to flavors, textures, and aromas. This practice not only enhances the enjoyment of food but also supports healthy digestion and prevents overeating. Imagine sitting down to a meal, free from distractions, fully appreciating the nourishment it provides.

Mindfulness also plays a crucial role in emotional healing, offering tools to navigate complex feelings and experiences. By observing emotions without attachment or aversion, individuals learn to respond rather than react, fostering emotional resilience and stability. This non-judgmental awareness creates space for healing and transformation, allowing individuals to process and release past traumas and negative patterns.

The practice of loving-kindness meditation, a form of mindfulness, cultivates compassion and empathy towards oneself and others. By silently repeating phrases of goodwill and love, individuals strengthen their capacity for kindness and connection, promoting emotional healing and well-being. Picture sitting quietly, envisioning a loved one, and sending them thoughts of peace and happiness, feeling the warmth of connection and compassion radiate within.

Mindfulness can be particularly beneficial in managing chronic pain, offering a complementary approach to traditional pain management techniques. By shifting focus from pain to the breath or other sensations, individuals can reduce the perception of pain and increase tolerance. This mindful approach empowers individuals to take an active role in their healing journey, fostering a sense of control and empowerment.

Stress, a common adversary in modern life, can be effectively mitigated through mindfulness practice. By cultivating a state of awareness and acceptance, mindfulness reduces the physiological impact of stress, lowering blood pressure, heart rate, and cortisol levels. This stress reduction promotes physical healing and enhances the body's ability to repair and regenerate.

The role of mindfulness in healing extends beyond the individual, influencing relationships and communities. As individuals cultivate mindfulness, they become more present and attentive in their interactions, fostering deeper connections and understanding. This ripple effect enhances collective well-being, creating a more compassionate and harmonious society.

Integrating mindfulness into daily life requires commitment and practice. Setting aside time each day for mindfulness exercises, whether through meditation, mindful movement, or simply being present in the moment, establishes a foundation for healing and growth. Even a few minutes of mindfulness practice can have a significant impact, offering a moment of peace and clarity in a busy day.

As individuals embrace mindfulness, they embark on a journey of self-discovery and healing, uncovering the richness and beauty of the present moment. This practice nurtures the mind, body, and spirit, fostering resilience, compassion, and well-being. By incorporating mindfulness into daily life, individuals unlock the potential for profound healing and transformation, creating a life of balance, harmony, and joy.

Cultivating a Positive Relationship with Food

Food is an integral part of our lives, serving not only as nourishment but also as a source of comfort, pleasure, and cultural identity. Cultivating a positive relationship with food is essential for overall well-being, allowing us to embrace the joys of eating while making mindful and healthful choices. By shifting our perspective on food, we create a balanced and harmonious relationship that enhances both physical and emotional health.

The foundation of a positive relationship with food begins with self-awareness and acceptance. Recognizing personal attitudes and beliefs about food allows individuals to identify any negative patterns or misconceptions that may be influencing their eating habits. For instance, Sarah, a young professional, realized she often associated guilt with eating dessert. By acknowledging this feeling, she began to question its origin and work towards a healthier mindset, allowing herself to enjoy sweets in moderation without remorse.

Mindful eating is a powerful practice that encourages individuals to engage fully with the eating experience. By slowing down and paying attention to the flavors, textures, and aromas of food, we can appreciate each bite and develop a deeper connection with our meals. This practice not only enhances enjoyment but also supports better digestion and hunger awareness. Imagine sitting at a table, taking a moment to savor the rich aroma of a homemade soup, feeling gratitude for the nourishment it provides.

Understanding the body's hunger and satiety signals is crucial for developing a balanced relationship with food. Learning to differentiate between physical hunger and emotional cravings empowers individuals to respond appropriately to their body's needs. By tuning in to these signals, we can avoid overeating and make more informed food choices. Picture yourself pausing before a meal, assessing your hunger level, and deciding to serve a portion that satisfies rather than overwhelms.

A positive relationship with food also involves embracing variety and flexibility in our diets. Enjoying a wide range of foods not only ensures nutritional completeness but also prevents monotony and deprivation. By allowing for occasional indulgences and maintaining a flexible approach to eating, we can enjoy the pleasures of food without guilt or restriction. Consider the excitement of trying a new cuisine or experimenting with an unfamiliar ingredient, each experience broadening culinary horizons and enriching the palate.

Food is deeply intertwined with culture and tradition, offering a sense of identity and belonging. Celebrating cultural heritage through food fosters a positive connection to our roots and creates opportunities for meaningful experiences with family and community. Reflect on the joy of preparing a traditional holiday dish, the kitchen filled with the laughter of loved ones and the aroma of familiar spices, each bite a taste of cherished memories.

Developing a positive relationship with food also involves cultivating gratitude for the journey from farm to table. Understanding the efforts of farmers, producers, and cooks instills a sense of appreciation and respect for the food we consume. This perspective encourages mindful consumption and reduces waste, fostering a sustainable relationship with the environment. Imagine visiting a local farmers' market, meeting the people who grow your food, and feeling a connection to the land and its bounty.

Emotional eating is a common challenge that can disrupt a positive relationship with food. Recognizing and addressing the emotions that drive eating habits is essential for making mindful choices. By finding alternative coping mechanisms, such as engaging in physical activity or practicing relaxation techniques, individuals can manage emotions without turning to food for comfort. Picture yourself taking a walk in the park, the fresh air and movement offering solace and clarity, rather than reaching for that extra serving of ice cream.

Building a supportive food environment is another key element in fostering a healthy relationship with food. Surrounding oneself with nourishing options and minimizing temptations creates a space that encourages mindful eating. Organizing the kitchen with nutritious staples and preparing meals at home more often can lead to healthier choices. Envision a pantry stocked with whole grains, legumes, and fresh produce, each ingredient an invitation to create wholesome and satisfying meals.

For parents and caregivers, modeling a positive relationship with food is crucial in shaping children's attitudes and behaviors. Encouraging children to explore different foods and involving them in meal preparation fosters curiosity and a sense of ownership over their eating habits. By demonstrating mindful and balanced eating, adults can instill lifelong healthy habits. Imagine cooking with a child, their eyes wide with wonder as they chop vegetables or stir a pot, each moment an opportunity for learning and bonding.

Developing a positive relationship with food is an ongoing journey that requires patience and self-compassion. Accepting that there will be challenges and setbacks allows individuals to approach the process with kindness and resilience. By reframing food-related experiences as opportunities for growth rather than failures, we cultivate a mindset that supports lasting change. Picture yourself reflecting on a day of eating, acknowledging both the choices that aligned with your goals and those that didn't, and feeling empowered to continue your journey with renewed commitment.

Ultimately, cultivating a positive relationship with food enriches our lives, allowing us to enjoy the pleasures of eating while nurturing our bodies and minds. By embracing mindfulness, variety, and gratitude, we transform food from a mere necessity into a source of joy, connection, and nourishment. As we develop this relationship, we unlock the potential for enhanced well-being, creating a life of balance and fulfillment.

Techniques for Mindful Meal Preparation

Mindful meal preparation is an art that transforms cooking into a meditative practice, enriching both the culinary process and the dining experience. It invites individuals to engage fully with the task at hand, fostering a sense of presence and awareness that permeates the food we prepare and consume. By adopting mindful techniques in the kitchen, we create meals that are not only delicious but also nourishing for the mind and body.

One key aspect of mindful meal preparation is setting the tone in the kitchen environment. Creating a space that is calm and inviting encourages focus and intentionality in the cooking process. Consider the atmosphere: perhaps you dim the lights slightly, open a window for a gentle breeze, or play soft music that soothes the senses. This environment sets the stage for a mindful experience, allowing you to immerse yourself in the rhythm of cooking.

Organizing ingredients and tools before beginning to cook, often known as mise en place, is a practice that embodies mindfulness. By arranging everything neatly and within reach, you minimize distractions and interruptions, allowing for seamless flow and concentration. Picture your cutting board surrounded by vibrant vegetables, each one washed and ready to be transformed into a delicious meal. This preparation is not just practical; it grounds you in the present moment.

Engaging the senses is central to mindful cooking. Feel the texture of the ingredients as you slice through a crisp apple or knead a soft dough. Notice the colors that brighten your workspace, from the deep green of spinach to the fiery red of bell peppers. Listen to the rhythmic chopping of a knife or the gentle sizzle of onions in a pan. These sensory experiences anchor you in the here and now, turning each step into a meditative act.

Mindful meal preparation also involves being present with your thoughts and emotions as you cook. Acknowledge any feelings that arise, whether they are joy, frustration, or nostalgia, without judgment or distraction. Allow these emotions to flow through you, observing them as part of the culinary journey. This awareness fosters a deeper connection with the food you prepare, infusing it with intention and care.

A gentle focus on the breath can enhance mindfulness in the kitchen. As you move through tasks, take a moment to breathe deeply, inhaling the aromas of fresh herbs or simmering spices. This practice cultivates calmness and clarity, allowing you to approach cooking with a centered and peaceful mindset. Imagine the soothing rhythm of your breath guiding you through each step, creating a harmonious dance between body and mind.

Mindful meal preparation encourages gratitude for the ingredients and their origins. Reflect on the journey each item has taken to reach your kitchen, from the farmer's field to your hands. This gratitude deepens your appreciation for the food and the effort involved in its production, fostering a sense of connection to the larger food system. Envision the hands that harvested your vegetables, the land that nurtured them, and the sun that ripened the fruits, each element contributing to the meal you are about to create.

Incorporating mindfulness into cooking techniques enhances the transformative power of the culinary process. When chopping vegetables, focus on the precision and rhythm of each cut. As you stir a pot of soup, feel the resistance of the spoon against the thickening broth. These actions, performed with attention and care, become meditative practices that center and ground you.

Mindful meal preparation can also involve mindful eating, a complementary practice that completes the cycle of awareness. Once your meal is ready, take a moment to sit quietly, free from distractions, and appreciate the colors, textures, and aromas before you. As you eat, savor each bite, noticing the flavors that unfold on your palate. This mindful approach to eating not only enhances enjoyment but also supports digestion and satiety, allowing you to listen to your body's needs and cues.

Sharing the experience of mindful meal preparation with others can deepen its impact and create lasting memories. Invite friends or family to join you in the kitchen, each person contributing to the process with their unique skills and perspectives. This communal activity fosters connection and collaboration, transforming meal preparation into a shared ritual of mindfulness and togetherness. Picture the laughter and camaraderie as you work side by side, each person fully present and engaged in the moment.

Mindful meal preparation is a journey that evolves with practice and intention. It invites us to slow down, appreciate the present, and cultivate a deeper connection to the food we prepare and consume. By embracing mindfulness in the kitchen, we transform cooking into a meaningful and fulfilling practice that enriches our lives and nourishes our souls. Through this mindful approach, we create meals that are not only sustenance for the body but also a source of peace and joy for the spirit.

Printed in the USA
CPSIA information can be obtained
at www.ICGtesting.com
CBHW070843031024
15215CB00094B/3265